THE SKILLS OF
COMMUNITY
SERVICE
COORDINATION

THE SKILLS OF COMMUNITY SERVICE COORDINATION

PSYCHIATRIC REHABILITATION PRACTICE SERIES : book 6

Mikal R. Cohen, Ph.D.
Director of Training, Center for Rehabilitation Research
    and Training in Mental Health
Research Associate Professor
Department of Rehabilitation Counseling
Sargent College of Allied Health Professions
Boston University

Raphael L. Vitalo, Ph.D.
Director, Consultation and Education
Springfield Community
Mental Health Consortium
Springfield, Massachusetts

William A. Anthony, Ph.D.
Director, Center for Rehabilitation Research and
    Training in Mental Health
Associate Professor
Department of Rehabilitation Counseling
Sargent College of Allied Health Professions
Boston University

Richard M. Pierce, Ph.D.
Director of Training Services
Carkhuff Institute of Human Technology
Amherst, Massachusetts

University Park Press
Baltimore

UNIVERSITY PARK PRESS
International Publishers in Science, Medicine, and Education
233 East Redwood Street
Baltimore, Maryland 21202

This book was developed by the Carkhuff Institute of Human Technology, 22 Amherst Road, Amherst, MA 01002, pursuant to Public Health Service Grant No. T21 MH 14502-20 with the National Institute of Mental Health; Alcohol, Drug Abuse, and Mental Health Administration, Department of Health, Education and Welfare.

THE PSYCHIATRIC REHABILITATION PRACTICE SERIES

Instructor's Guide
by *William A. Anthony, Ph.D.,*
Mikal R. Cohen, Ph.D., and Richard M. Pierce, Ph.D.

Book 1: **The Skills of Diagnostic Planning** / *William A. Anthony, Richard M. Pierce, Mikal R. Cohen, and John R. Cannon*
Book 2: **The Skills of Rehabilitation Programming** / *William A. Anthony, Richard M. Pierce, Mikal R. Cohen, and John R. Cannon*
Book 3: **The Skills of Professional Evaluation** / *Mikal R. Cohen, William A. Anthony, Richard M. Pierce, Leroy A. Spaniol, and John R. Cannon*
Book 4: **The Skills of Career Counseling** / *Richard M. Pierce, Mikal R. Cohen, William A. Anthony, Barry F. Cohen, and Theodore W. Friel*
Book 5: **The Skills of Career Placement** / *Richard M. Pierce, Mikal R. Cohen, William A. Anthony, Barry F. Cohen, and Theodore W. Friel*
Book 6: **The Skills of Community Service Coordination** / *Mikal R. Cohen, Raphael L. Vitalo, William A. Anthony, and Richard M. Pierce*

Library of Congress Cataloging in Publication Data
Main entry under title:

The skills of community service coordination.
   (Psychiatric rehabilitation practice series; book 6)
   Bibliography: p.
   1. Mentally ill—Rehabilitation. 2. Community mental health services. I. Cohen, Mikal R.
II. Series.
[RC439.5.S55]   362.2'0425   79-29693
ISBN 0-8391-1575-X

THE SKILLS OF COMMUNITY SERVICE COORDINATION ▮

CONTENTS

ABOUT THE AUTHORS

Dr. Mikal R. Cohen is the Director of Rehabilitation and Mental Health Services at the Carkhuff Institute of Human Technology, a non-profit organization dedicated to increasing human effectiveness. Dr. Cohen has been a practitioner in several outpatient and inpatient mental health settings, and has served as an administrator, inservice trainer, program evaluator and consultant to numerous rehabilitation and mental health programs. She has developed teaching curricula and taught the skills of psychiatric rehabilitation to practitioners throughout the United States. Furthermore, Dr. Cohen has authored a number of books and articles in the fields of mental health and health care.

Dr. Raphael L. Vitalo is Director of Consultation and Education at the Springfield Community Mental Health Consortium. Dr. Vitalo has experience in the development, implementation, coordination and evaluation of a broad range of programs serving psychiatric clients.

He has had responsibility for the provision of services including: outpatient, inpatient, alcoholism and drug abuse, follow-up, screening, emergency services, services to seniors and children, and supervision of partial hospitalization services. Dr. Vitalo is also the author of more than sixteen professional publications in the areas of treatment and mental health administration.

Dr. William A. Anthony is an Associate Professor and Director of Clinical Training in the Department of Rehabilitation Counseling, Sargent College of Allied Health Professions, Boston University. Dr. Anthony has been Project Director of a National Institute of Mental Health grant designed to develop and evaluate training materials for persons studying and practicing in the field of Psychiatric Rehabilitation. Dr. Anthony has been involved in the field of Psychiatric Rehabilitation in several different capacities. He has researched various aspects of psychiatric rehabilitation practice and has authored over three dozen articles about psychiatric rehabilitation which have appeared in professional journals.

Dr. Richard M. Pierce is Director of Training Services at the Carkhuff Institute of Human Technology, a non-profit organization dedicated to increasing human effectiveness. Dr. Pierce has extensive counseling experience and has consulted to dozens of local, state and federal human service programs. He has taught the skills and knowledge of psychiatric rehabilitation to practitioners from a variety of disciplines. Dr. Pierce is noted for his research on the training of counselors. Dr. Pierce has authored eight books and dozens of articles in professional journals.

CARKHUFF INSTITUTE of HUMAN TECHNOLOGY

The Carkhuff Institute of Human Technology is intended to serve as a non-profit international center for the creation, development and application of human technology. The Institute, the first of its kind anywhere in the world, takes its impetus from the comprehensive human resource development models of Dr. Robert R. Carkhuff. Using these models as functional prototypes, the Institute's people synthesize human experience and objective technology in the form of a wide range of specific programs and applications.

We live in a complex technological society. Only recently have we begun to recognize and struggle with two crucially important facts: improperly used, our technology creates as many problems as it solves; and this same technology has been delivered to us with no apparent control or "off" buttons. Our attempts to retreat to some pretechnological, purely humanistic state have been both foolish and ill-fated. If we are to develop our resources and actualize our real potential, we must learn to grow in ways which integrate our scientific and applied knowledge about the human condition with the enduring human values which alone can make our growth meaningful.

We cannot afford to waste more time in fragmentary and ill-conceived endeavors. The next several decades — and perhaps far less than that — will be a critical period in our collective history. Recognizing this, the Carkhuff Institute of Human Technology is dedicated to fostering the growth and development of personnel who can develop, plan, implement and evaluate human resource development programs while making direct contributions to the scientific and technological bases of these same programs. Thus the Institute's fundamental mission is to integrate full technical potency with fully human and humane goals — in other words, to deliver skills to people which let them become effective movers and creators rather than impotent victims.

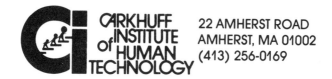

CARKHUFF INSTITUTE of HUMAN TECHNOLOGY

22 AMHERST ROAD
AMHERST, MA 01002
(413) 256-0169

PSYCHIATRIC REHABILITATION PRACTICE SERIES

PREFACE

This text is one of a series of six books designed to facilitate the teaching of various psychiatric rehabilitation skills. It is written for professionals practicing in the field as well as for students studying in such professions as nursing, rehabilitation counseling, occupational therapy, psychology, psychiatry, and social work. Each of these disciplines has contributed and will continue to contribute practitioners, researchers, administrators, and teachers to the field of psychiatric rehabilitation.

This series of training manuals evolved from a lengthy analysis of the practitioner skills that seemed to facilitate the rehabilitation outcome of persons with psychiatric disabilities. Under the sponsorship of the National Institute of Mental Health, each of these training manuals was developed and then field-tested on a group of rehabilitation mental health professionals and students. Based on the feedback of the training participants after the use of these skills with psychiatrically disabled clients, each training manual was revised. Thus, the content of the books reflects not only the authors' perspectives, but also the ideas of the initial group of training participants.

The ultimate purpose of this six-volume series is to improve the rehabilitation services that are presently offered to the psychiatrically disabled person. This training text is written for those practitioners whose rehabilitation mission is either: (1) to assist in the reintegration of the psychiatrically disabled client into the community; or (2) to maintain the ability of the formerly disabled client to continue functioning in the community and, in so doing, to prevent a reoccurrence of psychiatric disability. In other words, depending upon a client's particular situation, psychiatric rehabilitation practitioners attempt either to reduce their clients' dependence on the mental health system or maintain whatever level of independence the clients have already been able to achieve.

This mission can be accomplished when the focus of the psychiatric rehabilitation practitioner's concern is increasing the *skills* and *abilities* of the psychiatrically disabled client. More specifically, the rehabilitation practitioner works to promote the client's ability to employ those skills necessary to live, learn, and/or work in the community. Success is

i

achieved when the client is able to function in the community as independently as possible.

Historically, the primary focus in psychiatric rehabilitation has been on the development of alternative living, learning, and working environments. In such environments, psychiatrically disabled clients have been provided settings in which they can function at a reduced level of skilled performance that is still higher than the level of functioning typically demanded in an institutional setting. In addition, these rehabilitation settings have provided a more humane, active, and "normal" environment within which clients can function. The hope has been that, over a period of time, the more positive environment of these rehabilitation settings might help many clients to improve their ability to function more independently and, in many cases, to actually leave the rehabilitation setting.

Within the last decade, however, rehabilitation has come to involve much more than the development, administration, and coordination of specific settings. Psychiatric rehabilitation practitioners can now assume a direct rehabilitation role by *diagnosing critical skill deficits* in their clients and *prescribing rehabilitation programs* designed to overcome these skill deficits. The development of rehabilitation settings that emphasize the skills and abilities of the clients has helped lay the foundation for this approach to psychiatric rehabilitation.

Although the greatest boon to rehabilitation within the mental health system has been the development of new and unique environmental settings as alternatives to institutional living, the most significant failure of psychiatric rehabilitation has been its inability to train the psychiatric rehabilitation practitioner thoroughly in rehabilitation skills. Professionals from a wide range of disciplines (e.g., counseling, nursing, psychiatry, social work, and psychology) engage in the practice of psychiatric rehabilitation. For the most part, however, these various disciplines have only the expertise developed in their own professions to bring to the field of psychiatric rehabilitation. Their training has lacked a specific set of rehabilitation skills to complement the expertise of their own disciplines.

The present series of psychiatric rehabilitation training texts, of which this volume is a part, is designed to help overcome the lack of specialized training in psychiatric rehabilitation. These training books focus on the specific skills areas that are designed to equip the psychiatric rehabilitation practitioner with the expertise necessary to promote the abilities of the psychiatrically disabled client, either by increasing the client's skills and by modifying the environment so as to better accommodate the client's present level of skilled behavior.

The first two training books help the psychiatric rehabilitation practitioner to become more proficient in *diagnosing* and *teaching* the skills that the client needs to function more effectively in the community. The third book provides the practitioner with the skills necessary to *evaluate* the outcome of her or his rehabilitative efforts. Training books four and five focus specifically on practitioner skills that have been the traditional concern of the rehabilitation practitioner — *career counseling* and *career placement* skills. The sixth training book focuses on ways in which the rehabilitation practitioner can *use the resources of the community* to better accommodate the client's present abilities and programming needs.

Although each text is part of a series of training books, each has been designed so that it may be used independently of the other. The six books included in the series are:

1. **The Skills of Diagnostic Planning**
2. **The Skills of Rehabilitation Programming**
3. **The Skills of Professional Evaluation**
4. **The Skills of Career Counseling**
5. **The Skills of Career Placement**
6. **The Skills of Community Service Coordination**

The skills-learning *process* within the training books involves an explain-demonstrate-practice format. That is, the practitioner is first explained the skill, is then shown examples of the skill, and finally is provided with suggestions on how to practice or do the skill. The practice suggestions include first practicing in a simulated situation and then actually performing the skill with a psychiatrically disabled client.

The first chapter of each training book overviews the specific practitioner skills that comprise that text. The next several chapters of each text are the teaching chapters and present the explain-demonstrate-practice steps involved in learning each specific skill. The final chapter of each book suggests ways in which the practitioner can evaluate one's own or another person's performance of these skills. The reference section of the books contains the major references that are sources of further discussion of various aspects of the skills.

Each of the major teaching chapters has a vignette at the beginning and end of the chapter. This vignette or short story is designed to illustrate unsuccessful and successful applications of the specific skills that are the focus of that particular chapter. Its purpose is to give the reader an overview of the skills that are presented in each chapter. In addition, a summary of the skill behaviors that comprise each major skill is given at the end of each chapter section.

Each chapter contains practice suggestions for each skill that can facilitate the learners' practice of their newly developing skills. Often the learner is first asked to practice and demonstrate her or his skill learning by filling out some type of table or chart. These charts can serve as an observable demonstration of the learner's mastery of a particular skill. Most of these various charts are not needed in the day-to-day application of these skills with actual clients. However, during the skill-learning process, these charts or tables are useful in demonstrating the learner's present level of skill mastery, either to the learner her or himself or to the learner's supervisors and teachers.

The skill-learning *outcome* of each of these training volumes is an observable, measurable cluster of practitioner skills. These skills are not meant to replace the skills of the various disciplines currently involved in the practice of psychiatric rehabilitation; rather, these skills are seen as complementary to the professional's existing skills. The additional use of these rehabilitation skills can play an extremely important role in improving the efficacy of psychiatric rehabilitation.

The Psychiatric Rehabilitation Practice Series has developed out of the contributions of a number of different people. We are particularly indebted to a great many students and practicing professionals, who, by virtue of their willingness to learn these skills and provide knowledge as to their effectiveness, have allowed us the opportunity to develop, refine, and revise these texts.

We would also like to acknowledge the individual instructors who taught the first group of students from these texts, and gave willingly of their time and talents in the development of this series.

These initial instructors were Arthur Dell Orto, Marianne Farkas, Robert Lasky, Patrice Muchowske, Paul Power, Don Shrey and LeRoy Spaniol.

Particular appreciation is expressed to Marianne Farkas, who not only taught these skills, but who also assisted in the editing and evaluation of these training texts.

Boston, Massachusetts

W.A.A.
M.R.C.
R.M.P.

THE SKILLS OF COMMUNITY SERVICE COORDINATION

Chapter 1 THE COMMUNITY SERVICE COORDINATION MODEL

Stated most broadly, the goal of psychiatric rehabilitation is to restore to clients their capacity to function in the community. Philosophically, this means that rehabilitation is directed at increasing the *strengths* of the clients so that they can achieve their maximum potential for independent living and meaningful careers. Although many traditional treatment approaches seek to prepare clients to function independently, the emphasis in traditional psychiatric treatment has typically been on the reduction of client discomfort by changing underlying personality structures, increasing client insights, and alleviating symptomatology.

Although the total treatment process for disabled psychiatric clients includes aspects of both traditional psychiatric treatment and psychiatric therapy and rehabilitation, it is important that these activities be separated conceptually so that the rehabilitation process receives the emphasis necessary to develop its own unique contribution to client care.

This text represents one of a series of books whose purpose is to define and teach the unique skills of psychiatric rehabilitation. The particular skill with which this book is concerned is *community service coordination*.

THE DEFINITION, PURPOSE, AND APPLICATIONS OF COMMUNITY SERVICE COORDINATION

WHAT COMMUNITY SERVICE COORDINATION IS

Community service coordination is a process of getting clients the help they need from the individuals, programs, and agencies in the community responsible for and able to provide that help. Community service coordination is sometimes understood as part of the *case management* function (Joint Commission on Accrediting Hospitals, 1976; Title XX Service Definitions, 1975). It incorporates the case management activities of linking, monitoring, and coordinating/advocating, and it builds on the case management functions of assessment and planning. Specifically, community service coordination involves three specific steps: (1) selecting the appropriate community resource, (2) arranging for the client's utilization of the preferred resource, and (3) supporting the client's utilization of the resource.

WHY COMMUNITY SERVICE COORDINATION IS IMPORTANT

Community service coordination enables the rehabilitation practitioner to assist a client in finding help for needs that the practitioner does not directly serve. It equips the practitioner with the skills to utilize the services provided by community agencies and thereby to assist clients who need to gain access to such agencies. Community service coordination enables practitioners to avoid assuming direct care in areas where they are not sufficiently trained or areas in which they do not have the needed resources. A practitioner skilled in community coordination can successfully use other community care providers who are specifically trained to service those client needs and have the necessary resources.

Rehabilitation clients tend to experience a variety of problems in a variety of areas. For example, a particular client may be experiencing difficulty in the area of work adjustment. Frequently, a comprehensive assessment of the client will reveal additional problems that are contributing to the client's inability to establish full independent living. These problems may be in the living area and may include such difficulties as fulfilling role expectations within family relationships or meeting basic living needs (food, shelter, clothing, security). The problems may emerge within the community setting and may involve experiences of alienation and abuse through discrimination, racism, and sexism. The problems could also involve the learning area and relate to the client's ability to acquire the knowledge and skills necessary for independent living.

The overall impact of these problems is to reduce the client's capacity to succeed in specific areas as well as in the general mission of asserting independence. This situation of multifaceted problems is intensified in clients who experience a chronic disability and extended periods of psychiatric hospitalization. The capacity of such clients to deal with their problems is reduced by extended periods of exclusion from the community and from the tasks of maintaining independent living. Thus, clients who experience chronic disability and are frequently removed from the tasks of daily living have a greater need for resources to assist them in dealing with their problems.

No practitioner or rehabilitation agency can meet all the needs of all clients. Expertise in community service coordination allows a practitioner to respond to a variety of client needs. By facilitating the client's access to and use of other community resources, practitioners can build on what they themselves can directly provide and thereby make a more complete response to the client. Community service coordination maximizes the client's receipt of support in eliminating the variety of deficits that hinder achievement of the rehabilitation goal. It expands the client's community support system by successfully linking the clients to an array of resources that can be reutilized as the need arises. The experience of being connected to an extensive support system mitigates the client's sense of isolation and reduces stress. Finally, contact with practitioners skilled in community service coordination increases the likelihood that the entire range of the client's problems will receive attention.

Clearly, the skills of community service coordination are essential to the successful provision of service to clients. However, research suggests that simply being aware of client needs and making referrals to meet these needs are not enough. Studies indicate that less than two-thirds of clients referred to other community resources and/or advised to contact other community resources actually follow through and make the initial contact (Wolkon, 1970). Research also suggests that, of those clients who do make initial contact with the community resource, approximately 40 percent fail to follow through to the first face-to-face interview, and some 50 percent drop out before the provision of service is completed. Finally, of those clients who sustain themselves in the use of the resources (and this might be no more than 21 percent of those identified as needing the resource), only about one-half or two-thirds report receipt of benefit from care. These statistics suggest that even when practitioners attempt to implement community service coordination, only 10 to 14 percent of their clients may find the benefits they require. This percentage is lower with black and Hispanic persons (Sue, McKinney, Allen, and Hall, 1974).

Although research analyzing the failure of community service coordination efforts is not complete, some understanding of the sources of failure has been developed (Vitalo, 1979). The sources of failure include: inappropriateness of the resource to the client's need; inaccessibility of the resource to the client; lack of sensitivity of the resource to the unique cultural and/or linguistic perspective of the client; lack of systematic efforts by the resource to engage the client in receipt of its services; lack of support from sources outside the resource to deal with such client problems as failure to understand the need for the resource, anxiety about the stigma attached to utilization of the resource, and anxiety about approaching the resource to receive benefits.

This book represents a model for community service coordination that addresses the apparent sources of failure of current efforts at community service coordination. The model described in this book personalizes the process of identifying, selecting, and providing access to community resources by beginning with the client's experience and incorporating the client's unique concerns. Additionally, the model acts on these principles of client involvement and personalized service coordination in a systematic manner. The systematic approach ensures that all the variables important to the proper identification of the community resource are incorporated in decision making. Further, the systematic approach ensures that all the potential problems that might impede the client's access to the resource are recognized and resolved. Finally, the systematic approach ensures that the practitioner follows through to support the client's utilization of the resource. In essence, this model is designed to eliminate the sources of failure currently experienced in community service coordination.

WHEN COMMUNITY SERVICE COORDINATION CAN BE USED

Community service coordination skills can be used at any point in the rehabilitation process when the practitioner cannot provide the services a client requires. As previously suggested, community service coordination is more important for clients who have experienced chronic disability and/or long-term psychiatric hospitalization.

Community service coordination is most critical where the practitioner's professional responsibilities are defined in terms of *case management* function rather than as direct provision of a treatment service meeting a specific client need. In this regard, community service coordination is essential for practitioners in emergency service programs who respond to clients in crisis and maximize community resources to support the client and reduce the level of crisis. Similarly, the practitioner who is responsible for discharge planning and follow-up of clients in inpatient and residential programs would have a high need for community service coordination skills. Finally, community service coordination skills are essential for vocational rehabilitation practitioners who need to coordinate a variety of community resources to meet the needs of clients attempting to establish or reestablish successful employment. To reiterate, community service coordination skills can be used at any time in the rehabilitation process. They can be used prior to, concurrently with, or after the rehabilitation process. The determining criterion is the point at which the practitioner is unable to provide the necessary service to a client and a plan needs to be developed and implemented to use a community resource.

THE STAGES AND SKILLS OF COMMUNITY SERVICE COORDINATION

This book will discuss in detail how community coordination is accomplished. This section will simply overview the process involved. Community service coordination requires the practitioner to proceed through three developmental stages: (1) selecting the appropriate community resource; (2) arranging for the client's utilization of the preferred resources; and (3) supporting the client's utilization of the resource.

The first stage, *selecting the appropriate community resource,* involves identifying the individual, program, or agency that can meet the client's needs in a manner responsive to the client's values and concerns. Selection is achieved through the following skills: (1) identifying the client's community resource need; (2) identifying the available community resources; (3) identifying viable community resource alternatives; (4) understanding the client's preferences and values; (5) researching the potential community resource alternatives; and (6) choosing the appropriate community resource.

The second stage, *arranging for the client's utilization of the preferred resource,* involves connecting the client to the preferred community resource. The skills include: (1) preparing to make the resource aware of the client's need; (2) obtaining the agreement of the resource to provide service; (3) finalizing the arrangements to utilize the resource; and (4) developing a program to utilize the resource.

The third stage, *supporting the client's utilization of the resource,* ensures that the resource utilization program is implemented. It ensures the successful culmination of the community service coordination process. The skills involved in supporting the client's utilization of the resource include: (1) developing time lines for action; (2) developing reinforcers to ensure action; (3) monitoring performance; and (4) modifying the program to improve its effectiveness.

The stages of community resource coordination and the skills they comprise are presented in Table 1. The entire process of community service coordination rests on an accurate diagnosis of the client's strengths and deficits. The skills of diagnostic planning are critical prior to effective community service coordination. Although these skills are not addressed in this book, the first book of this series, *The Skills of Diagnostic Planning,* provides a complete discussion of a functional assessment process. The remainder of this book will focus on the skills involved in community service coordination.

The successful implementation of community service coordination requires that the practitioner understand several basic principles. A paramount principle is *client involvement* in the process of community service coordination. The practitioner will want to ensure that the skill of community service coordination is placed fully in the service of the client, that the client is the beginning point and the end point for the implementation of the skill. Furthermore, the concept of client involvement does not mean that the practitioner simply keeps the client "in mind" or informed; rather, it means that the client's involvement in the entire process is active and ongoing. The participation of the client, both verbal and behavioral, determines the needs that require service, and the values and concerns of the client shape the decisions as to how the needs are to be met. Client involvement goes beyond participation. The client has the final say in the selection of the community resource to be used. It is the client, of course, who will be affected by the selection and who will be expected to follow through and utilize the resource. Client involvement is sustained throughout the entire process to the point that community service coordination becomes a partnership endeavor with the practitioner assuming responsibility for expertise in implementation but never acting unilaterally without attempting to involve

Table I. The Stages and Skills of Community Service Coordination

Stage I. Selecting the Appropriate Community Resource

Skills: A. Identifying the client's community resource need
   B. Identifying available community resources
   C. Identifying viable community resource alternatives
   D. Understanding the client's values and preferences
   E. Researching the potential community resource alternatives
   F. Choosing the appropriate community resource

Stage II. Arranging for the Client's Utilization of the Community Resource

Skills: A. Preparing to make the resource aware of the client's need
   B. Obtaining the agreement of the resource to provide service
   C. Finalizing the arrangements to utilize the resource
   D. Developing a program to utilize the resource

Stage III: Supporting the Client's Utilization of the Community Resource

Skills: A. Developing time lines for action
   B. Developing reinforcers to ensure action
   C. Monitoring performance
   D. Modifying the program to improve its effectiveness

the client. In this regard, the practitioner will want to encourage the client to implement as many steps in the process as possible.

Community service coordination cannot be effectively implemented unless the client's rights are fundamentally protected. These rights include the *right to privacy and confidentiality*. The practitioner will want to recognize these rights; he or she will not involve others in resolving the client's problems or provide information to others about the client without the client's written consent. Further, certain information requires special consent to be released. Specifically, information concerning alcohol or drug abuse requires release forms that are defined in federal regulations. The only legitimate suspension of the rights to privacy and confidentiality occurs in the instances of danger due to homicidal or suicidal tendencies. Hence, the sharing of information concerning the client is inappropriate without the client's written consent.

The practitioner will also want to clearly understand the goal of the community service coordination process. This understanding is critical because it defines the responsibility and follow-through incumbent upon the practitioner. Simply, the practitioner is working for the relief of the client's need. *Hence, the practitioner's responsibility continues until that relief is achieved.* Thus, the act of referral and placement in and of itself does not represent the termination of the community service coordination process. The practitioner follows through to ensure that the referral and placement result in the desired outcomes. The practitioner's responsibility includes: (1) following through to assess the resource's impact on the client; (2) advocating for the client with the resource to ensure that the impact is beneficial and in the client's area of need; and (3) recycling the entire process of community service coordination if the particular community resource cannot resolve the client's need.

Finally, it is also important that the practitioner understand that the community resource — whether it be an individual, a program, or an agency — has a responsibility to deliver on its mandates or missions. The purpose of community resources is to deliver on specific client needs. In some instances, the needs will be defined as opportunities or environments that allow a client to exercise skills and achieve advancement. In any case, it is important for the successful implementation of community service coordination that *the practitioner know the particular mandate or mission of each community resource with which she or he is working.* Only if the practitioner understands the resource's mandate or mission can she or he hold the resource accountable for delivering on that mandate or mission.

The remainder of this book provides the details related to the three community service coordination stages and the practitioner skills necessary to coordinate community services. The complexity of the community service coordination process will vary depending on the needs of the client and the community resources involved. It is important, however, that the practitioner master the skills necessary to deal with the most complex situation. In this way, the practitioner will possess the ability to deal with the entire range of coordination problems.

Practitioners who work with community service coordination problems function in a variety of different roles — for example, as diagnosticians, resource persons, decision makers, coordinators, advocates, negotiators, program planners, support persons, and/or monitors. The last table in this text (Table 51) shows how each of these functions relates to each of the separate community service coordination skills presented herein. It may be helpful to refer to this summary table as each of the various practitioner skills is introduced.

Chapter 2 SELECTING THE APPROPRIATE COMMUNITY RESOURCE ▪▪▪▪

SELECTING THE APPROPRIATE COMMUNITY RESOURCE: AN UNSKILLED APPROACH

It was a measure of the real progress that Alice had made that she no longer tried to deny what was obviously true. A month earlier, she would have rejected all of Jerry's efforts to personalize her deficits — which was, of course, precisely why Jerry had not attempted to do too much too soon. He had recognized quite early that he would have to move slowly and carefully if he wanted to keep Alice as an outpatient.

Now things were definitely improving. Alice was almost at the point where she could start looking for regular work again. Yet Jerry knew — and Alice now accepted the fact — that she really wouldn't be in a position to compete for jobs until she had developed some new skills. In particular, Alice's past work record indicated that she had a very hard time indeed demonstrating either dependability — getting to work on time, keeping absences down, completing assignments on time — or the capacity to get along with other people.

"I know it's a problem," Alice said now, grimacing a little at the thought of her own past employment history. "And I know I have to work on those things. But — well, how do you go about picking up things like dependability and getting along with others?"

Jerry understood her concern. Fortunately, he told her, there were a number of sheltered workshops operating in the area. By getting involved with one of these, Alice would have a chance to work toward specific goals in these important areas without having to deal with the intense pressure and competitiveness of the regular job market. Jerry went on to help Alice develop practical step-by-step programs to reach her several skill-related goals.

All well and good. Yet, having worked well with Alice up to this point, Jerry became overconfident and made a serious mistake.

"I've checked out the workshops that would be open to you. They all seem to have interesting programs," he told her. "And one of these workshops turns out to be right around the corner from where you're living."

"Really?"

"Uh-huh. So I went ahead and found out that there is an opening for you in their program. Unless you can see some problem, you'll be starting first thing Monday morning."

Alice didn't see any problem. (How could she, knowing little or nothing about this particular program?) She and Jerry worked out all the arrangements. The weekend came and went and, before she knew it, Monday morning had come and Alice was reporting to the workshop.

Her work, it turned out, involved sorting book covers. "You've got to be kidding! For a job like this, I could leave my brain at home!"

In fact, the work turned out to be even duller and more tedious than Alice had expected. For a few days she tried to stick to the step-by-step programs she and Jerry had worked out. But it was no good. She simply couldn't stand the monotony. On Friday morning she was an hour late getting to work, explaining her tardiness only by saying, "I overslept — sorry." On Monday morning, she didn't even bother to get out of bed. Shortly after eleven o'clock, the supervisor called her at home. Asked whether she was sick, Alice retorted, "Yeah, sick and tired! I quit!" and hung up the phone.

Alice was a difficult person to work with. Yet she had definitely been making progress. Things might have worked out for her if only Jerry hadn't taken the path of least resistance in getting her into a sheltered workshop setting. Jerry had failed to involve Alice in the process of selecting an appropriate community resource, and the only criterion he considered was which workshop was closest to Alice's home. He didn't consider the nature of the work itself. And because he failed to do so, his client didn't make it.

A simple mistake — but one with disastrous consequences for the client.

Selecting the appropriate community resource involves identifying which community resource will meet the needs of the client in a manner responsive to the client's values and concerns. In selecting the most appropriate community resource, the practitioner maximizes the chances of the client's needs being met.

As discussed previously, the process of community service coordination can fail at various stages. When the initial hurdle of contacting a community resource is overcome, the next most significant source of failure is the client's failure to use the resource. Characteristically, this failure reflects the inappropriateness of the service or the unacceptability of the manner, method, or context in which it is delivered. The practitioner's effort in working with the client to select the most appropriate resource helps to minimize the possibility of failure in the initial stages of community service coordination.

The process of selecting the appropriate resource occurs whenever more than one resource serving the client's particular needs exists within the community. Certain steps within the selecting process, however, can be useful even when only one choice exists.

A systematic resource selection process offers several advantages: (1) the process occurs objectively and therefore may be shared with the client and, indeed, wholly completed by the client; (2) the rationale for choosing the resource is fully articulated and therefore can support the client's motivation to follow through and convince the community resource of the appropriateness of serving the client; and (3) the procedure can accommodate a large number of alternatives and can tailor a choice in a manner uniquely responsive to the client.

Selecting the appropriate community resource involves six skills: (1) identifying the client's community resource need; (2) identifying available community resources; (3) identifying viable community resource alternatives; (4) understanding the client's values and preferences; (5) researching the potential community resource alternatives; and (6) choosing the appropriate community resource.

These skills and the related subskills are portrayed in Table 2. Selecting the appropriate resource is necessary whenever a community resource can meet a client need not directly provided for by the practitioner. The success of the selection is evaluated by assessing the appropriateness of the resource to the client's need and the acceptability of the resource to the client's preferences.

Table 2. The Skills and Subskills of Selecting the Appropriate Community Resource

---

I. **Identifying the Client's Community Resource Need**

    A. Identifying the client's problem
    B. Identifying the client's service goal
    C. Identifying the resources needed to achieve the service goal
    D. Identifying the resources needed from the community

II. **Identifying Available Community Resources**

    A. Locating and obtaining community resource listings
    B. Obtaining essential information on community resources
    C. Organizing community resource listings

III. **Identifying Viable Community Resource Alternatives**

IV. **Understanding the Client's Values and Preferences**

    A. Orienting the client to the exploration of values
    B. Eliciting client preferences for cost, availability, accessibility, and acceptability
    C. Identifying other client preferences
    D. Operationalizing the client's values and preferences

V. **Researching the Potential Community Resource Alternatives**

    A. Planning the research effort
    B. Implementing the research plan

VI. **Choosing the Appropriate Community Resource**

    A. Assessing the resource's conformity to the client's preferences
    B. Computing the resource's desirability
    C. Identifying the most desirable resource
    D. Recycling the decision-making efforts

IDENTIFYING THE CLIENT'S COMMUNITY RESOURCE NEED

Identifying the client's community resource need means knowing what kind of help the client requires that cannot be directly provided by the rehabilitation practitioner or the client. Identifying the client's community resource need provides a focus for the community service coordination effort. It tells both the client and the practitioner what kind of community services need to be sought out in order to successfully achieve the service goals that have been identified. Further, it facilitates organization of the rehabilitation effort by clarifying the client's and the practitioner's responsibilities in achieving specific service goals. Thus, knowing the client's community resource need facilitates identifying appropriate sources of assistance for the client.

The process of identifying the client's community resource need proceeds through the following skills: (1) identifying the client's problem; (2) identifying the client's service goal; (3) identifying the resources needed to achieve the service goal; and (4) identifying the resources needed from the community.

IDENTIFYING THE CLIENT'S PROBLEM

Identifying the client's problem means knowing what is keeping the client from achieving satisfaction in his or her living, learning, or working activities. The practitioner will want to list the difficulties the client is experiencing in his or her current or anticipated living, learning, or working environments. The process of problem identification is part of diagnostic planning. A comprehensive treatment of diagnostic planning is provided in Book 1 of this series: *The Skills of Diagnostic Planning*. Table 3 presents an inventory of typical client problems. The problems are organized according to living, learning, or working environments.

Table 3. Sample Client Problems

Environment	Problem
Living	Can't resolve conflict with landlord
	Lives in a cold apartment
	Can't keep apartment neat
	Can't control crying-yelling outbursts in apartment
Learning	Can't sustain attention during counseling sessions
	Can't accurately report feelings
	Can't spontaneously state wants and needs
	Can't effectively listen to counselor
Working	Unemployed
	Can't complete written job applications
	Can't present strengths in job interview

Practice Situations

As a practice exercise, using a format similar to Table 3, identify problems that you experience in your living, learning, or working environments. Typical problems might include the following: living environment — haven't enough money, haven't enough space in home, can't keep relationships smooth and conflict-free, can't keep up with household chores; learning environment — have no private space to study, have professors who aren't clear in their presentations, can't take adequate notes, can't control anxiety over exams; working environment — can't decide what job would be best, have a job that doesn't pay enough.

Next, list the typical problems of clients serviced by your agency or setting. Is there in fact a group of typical problems that clients present to your agency or setting?

IDENTIFYING THE CLIENT'S SERVICE GOAL

The second subskill in identifying the client's community resource need is to identify the client's service goal. The service goal is the reverse of the client's problem. A client problem such as "lack of shelter" would have as a service goal, "adequate shelter." Similarly, a client problem such as "can't control excessive drinking" would have as a service goal, "can eliminate excessive drinking." Table 4 provides an example of various client service goals.

13

Table 4. Sample Client Service Goals

Environment	Problem	Service Goal
Living	Can't resolve conflict with landlord	Can resolve conflict with landlord
	Lives in a cold apartment	Lives in a properly heated apartment
	Can't keep apartment neat	Can keep apartment neat
	Can't control crying-yelling outbursts in apartment	Can control crying-yelling outbursts in apartment
Learning	Can't sustain attention during counseling sessions	Can sustain attention during counseling sessions
	Can't accurately report feelings	Can accurately report feelings
	Can't spontaneously state wants and needs	Can spontaneously state wants and needs
	Can't effectively listen to counselor	Can effectively listen to counselor.
Working	Unemployed	Employed
	Can't complete written job applications	Can complete written job applications
	Can't present strengths in job interview	Can present strengths in job interview

Practice Situations

As a practice exercise, work with the problems you previously generated and provide a goal for each problem. Simply reverse the problem and turn it from a deficit to an asset. Also attempt to develop a list of common client service goals for clients of your particular setting.

A full mastery of problem identification and goal setting for individual clients requires study in the area of diagnostic planning. *The Skills of Diagnostic Planning* provides a thorough treatment of this important skill area.

IDENTIFYING THE RESOURCES NEEDED TO ACHIEVE THE SERVICE GOAL

Once the practitioner has diagnosed the client's specific problems and goals, the next subskill is to identify the resources the client needs to achieve the goal. The community resources needed by the client will be determined on the basis of the difference between what is needed for the client to achieve the service goal and what can be provided either by the client or by the practitioner directly.

Identifying the client's resource need proceeds through two subskills: (1) identifying what the client needs to be able *to do* to achieve the goal; and (2) identifying what the client needs *to have* to achieve the goal. Mr. Harry S. will provide an example.

Mr. S.'s main problem is loneliness; that is, he has no friends. The service goal that emerges from his problem is simply to establish friendships. The first step in identifying the resources needed for developing friendships is to consider what things the client has to have to achieve this goal. These may include an opportunity to meet people; activities in which to engage with people; sufficient money to spend in relating to people.

After the step of determining what the client needs to have to achieve the goal of establishing friendships has been considered, the next step is to consider what the client needs to be able to do in order to develop friendships. In this category might be the ability to initiate conversations; the ability to show understanding for other people's feelings; the ability to show understanding for people's ideas.

Table 5 organizes the resource needs for Harry S. The "have" resources that were identified (contacts with people, activities to engage in) and the "do" resources (ability to initiate conversations, ability to show understanding for other people's feelings) are appropriately categorized. Essentially, to achieve any service goal it would appear that a number of resources are required. Indeed, the process of cataloguing the resources required for any goal suggests that effectively working with a client requires an appreciation not only for the breadth of the client's problems but also for the potential depth of the assistance that may be required to relieve any one of those problems.

Table 5.   Resource Needs (Harry S.)

Client Problem	Service Goal	"Have" Resources	"Do" Resources
Lack of friendships	Friendships	Opportunity to meet people	Ability to initiate conversations
		Money to spend in relation to people	Ability to show understanding for another's feelings
			Ability to show understanding for another's ideas

15

Practice Situations

As a practice exercise in identifying "have" and "do" resources, focus on the client problem of "unemployment." The service goal identified for this problem is "employment." Now list the "have" resources required to obtain this goal. "Have" resources can be identified by thinking in terms of the people, places, things, activities, or opportunities a client needs to realize the goal. For example, one of the people resources that may be needed for the "employment" goal is positive references — people willing to speak well of the client's abilities.

Next, list the "do" resources that the client will require in order to achieve the goal of employment. The "do" resources refer to client skills or competencies. An aid in thinking about "do" resources is to consider competency in three skill areas: physical, emotional/interpersonal, and intellectual. A client will require physical skills specific to the job being sought as well as skills to find and obtain that position. An intellectual resource would be the ability to complete a job application form. An example of an emotional resource would be the ability to respond to questions in the job interview. After you have completed this exercise, check your answers with those provided in Table 6. In addition, take the most typical client problems and goals of your agency or setting, and develop a list of sample resource needs for your most common client goals.

Table 6. Sample Resource Needs for the "Employment" Goal

Client Problem	Service Goal	"Have" Resource Needs	"Do" Resource Needs
Unemployment	Employment	Positive references	Ability to write a letter of application
		Names of possible employers	Ability to identify potential employers
		Proper clothing for job interviewing	Ability to complete a job interview
		Money for job-seeking activities	Ability to present job-related strengths
		A completed résumé.	Ability to groom self appropriately.

IDENTIFYING THE RESOURCES NEEDED FROM THE COMMUNITY

Identifying the resources needed from the community means clarifying what resources neither the client nor the practitioner can provide directly. Once the resources required to achieve a service goal are identified, the step of determining which of those resources will need to be sought from the community is a simple one. Table 7 presents an example of resources needed from the community for the goal of employment. The previously developed list of resources required to achieve the service goal of employment is used, and the final step of identifying which of those resources are required from the community simply entails labeling those resources that the client can directly provide and those resources that the practitioner can provide. The remaining, unlabeled resources will need to be obtained from other sources. These other sources are generically termed *community resources*. As community resources, they incorporate all other people, programs, and agencies that exist in the community and that can actually or potentially provide the resources required by the client. They incorporate the client's family, neighbors, congregation or parish members, as well as whatever professionals exist within the community. Similarly, programs may extend from the yearly block party that might be held in the client's neighborhood to a highly professionalized program of day-care service. Thus, the concept of community resource is broadly defined to include both the client's natural support system and the human-service care systems established in the community.

Table 7. Sample Resources Needed from the Community

Problem	Goal	Resource Needs ("Have" and "Do")	Source
Unemployment	Employment	Positive references	
		Names of possible employers	
		Proper clothing for job interviewing	Client
		Money for job-seeking activities	Practitioner
		A completed résumé	Practitioner
		Ability to write a letter of application	Practitioner
		Ability to identify potential employers	
		Ability to complete a job interview	
		Ability to present job-related strengths	
		Ability to groom self appropriately	

Practice Situations

Refer to the previously developed list of common client problems and service goals for clients of your particular setting. Develop an overview of the typical community resource needs for the most common client service goals. Obtain this overview by constructing a chart similar to Table 7 for each of your setting's most frequent service goals. This exercise will produce a summary of the type of community resource needs most often encountered by your setting.

IDENTIFYING THE CLIENT'S COMMUNITY RESOURCE NEED: A SUMMARY

Goal: To identify the help the client requires from sources other than the client or the rehabilitation practitioner

1. Identify the client's problem (i.e., what is keeping the client from achieving satisfaction in his or her living, learning, or working environment).
2. Identify the client's service goal.
3. Identify the resources needed to achieve the service goal. Identify what the client needs to be able to *do* to achieve the goal. Identify what the client needs to *have* to achieve the goal.
4. Identify the resources needed from the community. Determine what resources neither the client nor the practitioner can directly provide.

IDENTIFYING AVAILABLE COMMUNITY RESOURCES

Once a client's community resource needs have been identified, the next skill is to identify the community resources available to meet the client's specific need. In order to help the client select the most appropriate resource, the practitioner develops a working knowledge of a number of community resources. In addition, the practitioner obtains new community resource information as the need arises. Knowing the available community resources enables the practitioner and the client to select the resource that appropriately meets the client's needs.

Identifying available community resources proceeds through three subskills: (1) locating and obtaining community resource listings; (2) obtaining essential information on community resources; and (3) organizing community resource listings. The outcome of this particular skill is an organized body of knowledge with respect to all the community resources that exist. Essentially, it allows the practitioner to develop a systematic, updated file of community resources. This text presents this particular skill at this point in the community service coordination model, but it is a skill that is used routinely by the practitioner so that her or his knowledge of available community resources is continually updated.

LOCATING AND OBTAINING COMMUNITY RESOURCE LISTINGS

In developing knowledge about various community resources, the practitioner's first task is to identify who has directories or catalogues of the community resources that exist within the service area. In any geographical area, a variety of programs and agencies develop listings of resources. Some of these programs and agencies do so as part of their own performance of monitoring and evaluation functions. Others develop lists to support their information and referral services. Still others develop lists for the purposes of soliciting members and developing directories for distribution. Although the resources being discussed are individuals, programs, agencies, and organizations available to a community, the practitioner will want to remember that clients have a unique resource system in the form of their natural support network. The client's natural support system consists of the people, places, things, and activities immediately connected to the client (e.g., relatives). This support system can be considered a valuable community resource.

A strategy to identify community resource listings involves determining: (1) who funds human service programs; and (2) who is responsible for referring large numbers of people with different problems to various programs. The practitioner can answer these questions by asking supervisors or administrators within the rehabilitation agency and by contacting the local United Way to see if it funds a centralized information and referral or hotline service. Additionally, if a federally funded community mental health center exists within the service area, it may be contacted to ascertain whether it provides centralized information and referral or hotline service.

Essentially, the funders of services maintain listings of the programs they fund and the purposes for which they are funded. Similarly, high-volume information and referral programs usually maintain up-to-date and comprehensive listings of community resources.

The practitioner's next step is to obtain copies of the community resource listings. This can be accomplished by obtaining the address and telephone number of the agencies that maintain centralized listings and identifying whom to contact.

Generally, the address and telephone number of specific agencies having centralized listings are available through the local telephone directory. Governmental agencies are listed under city, town, or state headings in the telephone directory. The local library should have in its reference section a listing of social service agencies as well as a listing of the local town, city, and state offices. Very commonly, the local

United Way publishes a social service directory providing listings that include addresses and telephone numbers and names of heads of programs for local human service providers, programs, and agencies.

Practice Situations

Table 8 presents a generalized list of sources for locating service listings. As a practice exercise, identify which of the resources listed in Table 8 exist in your community. Add to the list in Table 8 those resources in your community that possess lists of individuals, programs, and/or agencies providing services. In checking out the list provided in Table 8, you may wish to use both *people* and *written* sources. People sources would include colleagues at your agency or instructors at your university and the reference librarian at your local library. Written sources include the Yellow Pages of your local telephone directory; reference materials at your local library; newspapers; and service planning documents such as the state Title XX social service plan (State Department of Public Welfare) which are available to the public on request and contain the identification of providers of service throughout the localities within the state.

As a practice exercise, identify five of the generic resources listed in Table 8 that exist within your community and collect the information required to contact them for their listings of resources. Once you have collected this information, contact the person identified as the resource and arrange for access to any listing of resources they may have. To complete the access, you may need to actually go to the resource and make a copy of the listing, or you may be able to purchase a listing.

OBTAINING ESSENTIAL INFORMATION ON COMMUNITY RESOURCES

As information is obtained on a number of different resources, it is most efficient if the information is organized in a systematic and usable way. Obtaining the essential information on community resources involves identifying *what service* is provided *to whom* by that resource. Obtaining such essential information allows the practitioner to know whether a particular resource is relevant to a particular client in terms of both the client's need and the client's *eligibility*. In addition to the previously obtained information (name of agency, contact person, address, telephone number), the essential information includes: (1) services offered; (2) age level served; (3) geographical area served; (4) income level served; and other eligibility criteria. An example of information about a community resource is provided in Table 9.

As can be seen from the example, the information is "essential" in that it allows the practitioner and the client to quickly determine the relevancy of the resource. In this example, the agency and the service

Table 8. Locations of Community Resource Listings

Individual Resources

Client
Family members
Neighbors
Fellow association and club members
Fellow church members
Classified pages of telephone book under professional listings
Medical/Dental Bureau listing
Local Legal Aid Society (lawyers)
Local Medical Society (physicians)
Local Nurses' Registry (nurses)
Local Psychological Society (psychologists)
Local Social Workers' Association (social workers)

Programs/Agencies

Local church
Local school/university
Council of Churches
Department of Employment Security (state)
Department of Vocational Rehabilitation (state)
Department of Public Welfare (state)
Department of Public Health (state)
Area Council on Aging
Department of Youth Services (state)
Department of Mental Health (state)
United Way
Local federally designated community mental health center:
    (a) emergency service
    (b) coordinator for senior services
    (c) coordinator for children's services
    (d) coordinator for substances abuse
    (e) director of consultation and education
Local information and referral or help hotline
Local rape crisis hotline
Alcoholics Anonymous
Parents Anonymous
Parents without Partners
Recovery, Inc.
Salvation Army social service office
Catholic Charities and/or diocese office
Weight Watchers
Chamber of Commerce
Local Community Action Commission
Local Urban League
Local N.A.A.C.P.
City Department of Human Services
City Planning Office

offered are relevant only for people experiencing problems heating their residences and, more restrictively, to adults and seniors of a particular income level, residential area, and circumstance. Clearly, unless the client's need was in this area and the client conformed to the eligibility criteria, further consideration of this resource would be unnecessary.

Table 9. Sample Community Resource Information

Name of agency: _____ Council of Churches _____

Whom to contact for best results: _____ Rev. Ray Watts _____

Address: _____ 123 Front Street _____

Telephone: _____ 799-4721 _____

Services offered: _____ Emergency fuel assistance _____

Age level served: _____ 18+ years _____

Geographical area served: _____ City of Springfield _____

Income level served: _____ $8,500 and under for a family of four _____

Other eligibility information: _____ Problem must present danger to health; no other remedy possible _____

Practice Situations

Complete the essential information for two of the resources that you have identified in your community. Use a format similar to Table 9.

ORGANIZING COMMUNITY RESOURCE LISTINGS

The final subskill in identifying available community resources is to organize the community resource listings that have been obtained. The practitioner will want to organize the information so that it is usable, accessible, and related to the achievement of the service goals. Thus, the practitioner can list the identified community resources under headings representing the general client need areas. Table 10 provides a list of major client need areas.

The "need list" enables the practitioner to organize the resources that have been identified within the community. The format for organization may be determined by convenience. The practitioner may use file folders labeled with headings such as those contained in Table 10, in which the essential identifying information for the individuals, programs, and agencies providing for needs in the area is placed. Alternately, the practitioner may use a card index in a loose-leaf binder, again sectioned according to need areas and the resources providing services in these areas. The method selected should be flexible enough to allow for addition and deletion of resources, sturdy enough to hold up under use, and portable enough to be used by the practitioner and the client. The development of such a community resource file makes the practitioner her or himself an extremely helpful resource person. A current, organized file of resources is in and of itself a valuable resource.

Table 10.   Major Client Need Areas for Community Resources

Assistance in the area of:

Food
Shelter
Money
Housekeeping/home-repair services
Health/physical medical services
Transportation
Clothing
Emergency fuel assistance
Safety/protection from harm
Opportunities for socialization
Opportunity for recreation
Education and/or providing education
Information and referral for a variety of needs
Mental health emergency services
Mental health outpatient services
Mental health inpatient services
Alcohol abuse services
Drug abuse services
Services for the blind
Services for the mentally retarded
Job counseling assistance
Vocational retraining/rehabilitation services
Job placement services
Child day-care services
Services for the physically handicapped
Translation services
Self-help services
Legal assistance/consumer rights services
Advocacy groups' services
Tenant rights
Employment opportunities

Practice Situations

As an addition to the previous exercises completed in this section, assemble the sheets of essential identifying information you have compiled, and organize these sheets according to the categories in Table 10. A file-folder method may be most appropriate, because it will permit the greatest flexibility as you expand your collection of essential identifying information on more and more resources.

IDENTIFYING AVAILABLE COMMUNITY RESOURCES: A SUMMARY

Goal: To identify the community resources available to meet the client's need

1. Identify the programs or agencies that have dictionaries or catalogues of community resources.

2. Obtain copies of the community resource listings.

3. Complete the essential information on community resources.

4. Organize the community resource listings under headings representing client need areas.

IDENTIFYING VIABLE COMMUNITY RESOURCE ALTERNATIVES

At this point, the practitioner has completed two of the three skills involved in selecting an appropriate community resource: (1) identifying the client's community resource need; and (2) identifying the available community resources. The next skill is to be able to identify viable community resource alternatives for individual clients. In identifying viable community resource alternatives, the practitioner will want to consider all possible means of achieving the client's rehabilitation goal. Resources that do not relate to the client's need or goal and cannot be developed so that they would relate are eliminated from consideration. Also, resources that do provide services in the area of the client's need but have eligibility criteria that the client is unable to meet are eliminated from consideration. Fundamentally, then, *viable community resource alternatives are those programs that relate to the client's need and for which the client is eligible.* This includes agencies that may be persuaded to provide the service required by the client or to waive an eligibility criterion. Hence, when developing the specific alternatives, the practitioner is looking for individuals, programs, or agencies that can either actually or potentially provide the required service to the client.

In identifying viable community resource alternatives, the practitioner will want to (1) draw information from written sources and (2) draw information from people sources. Written sources can include the practitioner's resource file, whose development was previously discussed. Again, the file may be a new creation enriched by information from various clients, or it may be a modification of an existing list obtained from other sources. Additional written sources can include recent announcements distributed within the agency or mailed to the practitioner by other service providers, and local newpaper coverage of established or newly developed human service programs. The practitioner may want to add the information obtained from the written sources to the ongoing resource file to maximize its comprehensiveness and currency.

People sources of information may include colleagues, supervisory personnel, radio and/or TV advertisements, the staff of a local information and referral service or help hotline; the client; and other individuals involved with the client. Again, the essential information can be developed for the resources identified through people sources, and this information can be added to the practitioner's personal resource file.

An example of the process of identifying viable resource alternatives is the case of Mrs. King, who needs emergency fuel allocation. She has run out of fuel with which to heat her house and has no funds to purchase any. Mrs. King is a senior citizen, seventy years of age. She is female, black, and low-income (under $5,500 per year). She lives in the inner city. The absence of fuel represents a potential danger to Mrs. King's otherwise good health. A review of the resource file developed by her practitioner revealed that the Council of Churches provides an emergency fuel allocation program. In speaking with Mrs. King directly and in identifying the resources within her own natural support system, the practitioner learned that Mrs. King's children live close by and remain interested in and concerned about her welfare. A check with a staff colleague revealed that, in addition to the Council of Churches, the local Community Action Commission also provides an emergency fuel allocation program. Thus, three resources appear relevant to Mrs. King's need: the Council of Churches, Mrs. King's children, and the local Community Action Commission.

Having developed a list of actual or potential providers of service in the area of client's need, the practitioner will want to establish whether the client is eligible for these services. Again, eligibility can be assessed both in terms of the letter of the requirements and in terms of the possibility of special provision being extended. In assessing the client's eligibility, the practitioner will want to gather the essential information on each of the resource alternatives identified. The practitioner will also want to gather parallel information on the client. Thus, community resources that can provide the required service but do not extend the service to the population of which the client is a member would be eliminated at this point. Only those agencies that provide a service relevant to the client's need and provide it to the population to which the client belongs remain viable resource alternatives. Determinations, in most instances, will be made in terms of the following qualifying client characteristics: age, sex, income level, and geographical residence. By and large, eligibility criteria are written in these terms. Particular resources, however, may have unique eligibility criteria, of which the practitioner will want to be aware. Again, it is necessary to collect the essential information on each of the identified potential resources.

Once the essential information is identified for each of the potential resources, it is compared with the information for the client. If the client meets the characteristics of the target population of a particular resource, that resource is then considered a viable alternative.

Table 11 presents Mrs. King's conformity to the eligibility criteria of the three resources identified to meet her needs for emergency fuel allocation. Again, her need could be met by three identified resource alternatives: the Community Action Commission, the Council of Churches, and her children. The essential information on Mrs. King includes: age, seventy years; sex, female; income, under $5,500 per year; and residence, inner city. As it turns out, Mrs. King fulfills the eligibility criteria of each resource. If, however, Mrs. King could not meet the eligibility criteria of one of the resources and those criteria could not be waived, that resource would be eliminated from future consideration. In this instance, the practitioner would want to check back with the resource to determine if any exceptions are made. The practitioner might also want to obtain a copy of the bylaws and/or governmental regulations overseeing the operation of the resource since they may contain directives that would provide for the exemption from eligibility requirements.

Practice Situations

Return to your previous list of service goals, and select one of the service goals identified. Check the resource listing you have developed, and identify individuals, programs, or agencies that service that need. Once you have identified a list of potential resource alternatives, complete the task of gathering essential information so that you can assess a potential client's ability to meet the eligibility criteria. Your efforts should produce a table similar to Table 11.

Table 11. Conformity to the Eligibility Criteria of Alternative Community Resources (Mrs. King)

CLIENT DATA	COMMUNITY RESOURCES		

Client need: Emergency fuel allocation

	Community Action Commission	Council of Churches	Children
Age 70 years	Yes	Yes	N/A
Sex female	Yes	Yes	N/A
Income under $5,500/yr.	Yes	Yes	N/A
Residence inner city	Yes	Yes	N/A
Other	⎯	⎯	⎯
Appropriateness	Yes	Yes	N/A

IDENTIFYING VIABLE COMMUNITY RESOURCE ALTERNATIVES: A SUMMARY

Goal: To select the resources that relate to the client's rehabilitation goal and for which the client is eligible

1. Use brainstorming skills to identify actual or potential resource alternatives.

2. Gather essential information on each resource.

3. Gather parallel information on the client.

4. Compare the information to determine the client's eligibility.

UNDERSTANDING THE CLIENT'S VALUES AND PREFERENCES

The next major skill in selecting the appropriate community resource is to understand the client's values and preferences. A great part of the failure of community service coordination has been the failure of clients to follow though due to the lack of perceived relevance or acceptability of resources. All too often clients are not involved in the selection of the best community resource. The client's own value system is sometimes not even considered. Hence, an understanding of the client's values and preferences is critical in ensuring that the selected resource will be perceived as worthwhile by the client and increasing the likelihood of client follow-through.

Understanding the client's values and preferences can emerge organically from the rehabilitation relationship. That is, as the practitioner responds to the client and supports the client's sharing of experience, the practitioner will develop a picture of who the client is and how the client perceives his or her situation. Before implementing community service coordination skills, the practitioner will want to have a grasp of at least the most critical values and concerns of the client.

The subskills involved in the process of understanding the client's preferences and values include: (1) orienting the client to the exploration of values; (2) eliciting the client's preferences for the critical values of cost, availability, accessibility, and acceptability; (3) identifying other client preferences; and (4) operationalizing the client's values and preferences.

ORIENTING THE CLIENT TO THE EXPLORATION OF VALUES

The practitioner's first task is to prepare the client to participate in developing a picture of his or her preferences. Clients are able to participate more effectively in the process of rehabilitation when they are oriented to or prepared for their role. To prepare the client, the practitioner will want to explain three things: (1) what exploration of values is; (2) why it is important; and (3) what is expected of the client. An additional fourth step is to show the client what he or she is expected to do. This step may not need to be used with clients for whom explaining is sufficient. A demonstration can be accomplished by having the client listen to an audio/visual recording of a person role-playing the activities that are expected.

The following excerpt is an interaction between a practitioner and a client named Jane. The excerpt provides an example of orienting a client to the exploration of values:

Practitioner:	Jane, we have worked hard together over the past several sessions in identifying the problems and difficulties that are getting in the way of your establishing successful employment. And we have worked to find goals relative to each of those problems. We then organized these goals so that we could go at them one by one and increase our chances of being successful. The one that came up first for us was the goal of enabling you to relate to people in authority in your work settings more effectively. What we want to do is increase your skills in being able to establish and maintain positive relationships with those people so that the atmosphere on the job is comfortable rather than tense. How does that sound so far in terms of your picture of what we have been doing?
Client:	Well, that sounds pretty good to me. It has been a lot of work, but I am really feeling like maybe I can succeed on the job. I am really happy that I have been able to be a part of figuring all this out.
Practitioner:	In some ways, working on your problem with me has already given you a taste of success, and that's pretty thrilling.
Client:	Yeah! And we have gone further too. Using that resource catalogue you gave me, I was able to come up with some possible resources to help me learn those skills of dealing with authority. In fact, we got three. The local community mental health center outpatient department has a special communications group that focuses on authority. Then there was the course being provided by the community college in its adult education section on dealing with bosses. Then there was that special program offered by the Women's Task Force. That's not bad, I never thought we'd find three.
Practitioner:	Well, you worked hard, Jane. You searched around and contacted some people and did library research, and that made the difference. The fact that you found three resources means that now we have to choose among those three. We have to decide which one is the best one for you. An important part of that decision making is determining what your values or preferences are with respect to who can best assist you in developing the skills of dealing with people in

29

	authority. That is what I would like to do today with you. I'd like to explore with you your values and preferences. What that means is understanding what things are important to you about the program we get help from. It is important for us to do this because, unless the resource really suits you, you're not likely to draw benefit from it. How does that sound to you?
Client:	Sounds fine to me!
Practitioner:	What I would like you to do, Jane, is to think about what your concerns are in using a community resource to help you with learning these important skills — and to tell me what comes to mind. I'll work with you and raise some potential concerns that may help you in your thinking, but I don't want you to be limited to the issues that I come up with. Is this acceptable to you?
Client:	Sure. You know I have some concerns. As I was looking into the programs, some of what I found raised some questions, and I would like the opportunity to talk it over with you.

This example of orienting a client took place within the context of an ongoing rehabilitation relationship. In the example, the practitioner preceded the process of orienting the client with a review of what they had achieved to date. As a general rule, the practitioner will want to consolidate what has been achieved before moving ahead; consolidation serves as a base for what is to come next. The example continues with the practitioner introducing the task of identifying the client's preferences and providing a definition of what it is and why it is important and a description of how the client is expected to participate in that process.

Practice Situations

Think about how you would orient a client in a counseling situation, and write down what you would say. If you are studying the skill of community service coordination with others, share what you would say with fellow students. This exercise can broaden your perspective on how to introduce and orient a client to identifying preferences.

ELICITING CLIENT PREFERENCES FOR COST, AVAILABILITY, ACCESSIBILITY, AND ACCEPTABILITY

The next subskill in the process is to elicit the client's preferences for the critical values of cost, availability, accessibility, and acceptability. These four preference areas are critical because they frequently become barriers to care. Included in these four areas are such issues as cost, the presence of waiting lists, physical accessibility, the program's reputation, and its sensitivity to minority perspectives. Problems in any of these areas can limit the likelihood of the client's successful utilization of the resource. Hence, the practitioner will want to obtain the client's concerns about these issues. Once the client has explored these four value areas, the practitioner will then encourage the client to consider any other values the client thinks are important.

The following excerpt from the continued interaction between Jane and her practitioner provides an example of eliciting client preferences on the issues of cost, availability, accessibility, and acceptability.

Practitioner:	Well, Jane, I feel from our previous conversations that I already have an idea of what's important to you. I'd like to share that with you a little later, but first I'm wondering if we could look at some specific issues that frequently come up when a person is using another resource and around which people tend to have some concerns. Cost is the first of these. What would your thinking be about the issue of cost?
Client:	Well, this could be a real problem for me. You know I'm out of work right now. I've got a little money saved up, but I really need that for living.
Practitioner:	What you are saying, Jane, is that you are really pressed financially now and any cost would be a real burden for you.
Client:	Yeah. Any cost could be a real problem for me.
Practitioner:	Okay. We'll be looking into that a little more specifically in a few moments, but now I'd like to ask you about a general issue of availability. What I mean by availability is two things — like how quickly you can get the service, and what hours services are provided; also, anything else that has to do with the openness of services. Any concerns about availability?

Client:	Well, sure, I don't want to be waiting around. We've made a good start here, and I would want to try to build on it quickly. That would be real important to me. The hours don't much matter because right now I'm not working. If I get a job — then there would be a question. On the other hand, given the kind of problem I've got, it may be stupid for me to take a job now until I know I can do better than I've done before.
Practitioner:	Sounds to me, Jane, that you are saying that, concerning these two availability issues, getting into service quickly is the only real one for you. You are really anxious to act on the strength and confidence you have developed thus far. Sounds like you worry that if you wait too long you may lose some of that edge you have going for you right now.
Client:	Right! I never was rolling this good before, and I don't want to slow down!
Practitioner:	All right! How about the issue of accessibility? Accessibility includes where the service is located, whether the service facility has any physical barriers to its use by the handicapped, and so on.
Client:	Well — I don't have a car right now. I have to get there by some means of transportation or, if it's close enough, I can walk it. Otherwise, I don't know how I would get there.
Practitioner:	So any resources we use would have to be readily accessible by public transportation or be in walking distance from you. OK. The last issue I would like to ask you about is the question of acceptability. This is a big one that includes a lot of different matters. One that I think may have some special meaning for you has to do with the cultural sensitivity of the people at the resource. I guess we have to face it, and the facts are that blacks haven't always been received or served well in a lot of our community services and, as a black woman, this might be one of the concerns you'll have regarding acceptability. Other concerns people have are about the kind of methods a program uses or staff competence or the reputation of the program for being effective. Sometimes there are questions about the kind of setting in which services are offered. These are all issues concerning the area of acceptability.

Client:	Those are some heavy issues. I'll tell you right out I don't want to go any place where black people aren't wanted. I'm not dealing with that aggravation now. Now I'm dealing with getting myself together. I also want the place to have a good reputation. I don't want to run with losers. I don't care much about the setting, and as far as the approach they use goes, well, for sure, I want to learn something I can *use*. I don't want a lot of words. I want something that can help me be successful!
Practitioner:	You're really determined about the business of growing and achieving more for yourself, and you have no time to waste with anyone or anything that can't appreciate and contribute to that. So, agencies with hang-ups about blacks and programs that don't deliver real skills or don't have a reputation for delivering anything are not want you want.

As can be seen in the example, the content of exploration is predetermined, but the process is open and flexible in supporting the free expression of the client. The practitioner, therefore, will want to be proficient in the skills of demonstrating understanding and supporting exploration.

Practice Situations

Table 12 provides a list of specific issues for each of the major areas of cost, availability, accessibility, and acceptability. As an exercise, explore your feelings and thoughts about each issue. Write down your personal concerns regarding each of the issues, and give examples of how each might impact on your own community service coordination efforts.

In addition, think of a community resource that you yourself might be using in the future (e.g., an educational setting, a recreational setting). Identify your own specific preferences with respect to the values of cost, availability, accessibility, and acceptability.

Table 12.   Client Issues in Choosing the Most Appropriate Community Resource

Major Area	Client Issues
Cost	Charge for using the resource
Availability	Speed with which person can begin receiving service
	Availability of twenty-four-hour, seven-day-a-week emergency assistance
	Hours and days on which regularly scheduled services are offered
Accessibility	Proximity of resource to major transportation center
	Proximity of resource to client
	Accessibility of locality to physically handicapped
	Presence of staff who speak client's language
Acceptability	Reputation of resource for effectiveness
	Level of staff competence
	Sensitivity of resource to unique cultural perspectives and values of minorities
	Methodology and approach of resource
	Setting in which services are offered

IDENTIFYING OTHER CLIENT PREFERENCES

Once the practitioner has a picture of the client's concerns about specific issues, it is necessary to provide an opportunity for open-ended exploration to identify any remaining issues. This process ensures that all important matters are identified and incorporated within the decision making. The practitioner's understanding of the client's unique values and perspectives represents a beginning point for open-ended exploration. Thus, in the interaction below between Jane and her practitioner, the practitioner begins by sharing what had been learned about Jane thus far.

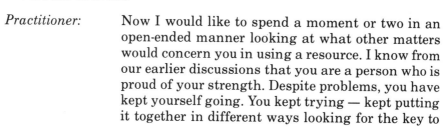

Practitioner: Now I would like to spend a moment or two in an open-ended manner looking at what other matters would concern you in using a resource. I know from our earlier discussions that you are a person who is proud of your strength. Despite problems, you have kept yourself going. You kept trying — kept putting it together in different ways looking for the key to success. I guess that tells me that you would want a program or a resource that would address your strengths. It tells me that you might want a resource with people who can recognize and give you credit for your strengths. How does that sound?

Client: Sounds fine! I think you're saying it. I don't want any downbeat program. I don't want any program that can't see me moving up and can't give me something to move up with. And I want the room to try on my own. That's the only way I'm going to know what's mine — what I've got to go with. You know — there are a lot of pressures on me. I'm a black woman. There are a lot of different ideas people have about a black woman, and all of them are traps. She is easy for sex. She can always get ahead because they are always ready to hire a black woman over a black man. She can always hold on to what she gets because nobody can go against a black woman and come out looking good. On the other hand, she never really wants anything but to be taken care of. It is all a bunch of garbage. And it all robs me of what I am. I guess if there is anything else I want from a resource, it is I don't want them tangling me up in those kinds of ideas. I want to be dealt with as me!

Practitioner: You're fed up with small people making more aggravation for you. You don't want to use a resource where the people you're going to have to deal with can't set aside their distortions and respond to you as you are.

Practice Situations

Building on the previous practice exercise, reflect on your unique concerns. List the things that are important to you and relevant to selecting a resource you might use (e.g., prestige, independence, friendships, recognition). Think about the experiences you've had that have given you an understanding of who or what works and/or doesn't work for you.

OPERATIONALIZING THE CLIENT'S VALUES AND PREFERENCES

As the client's values, concerns, and preferences are identified, they need to be *operationalized*. Operationalizing means to define, in an observable and measurable way, what is meant by each value. Unless the practitioner and the client precisely understand the value or concern, it cannot be used to make a decision. Often, in operationalizing a value, it becomes clear that what the practitioner thought the client meant was different from what the client really meant. Similarly, in operationalizing values, the client may readjust his or her perspective and arrive at a definition that differs from the initial definition. Values such as independence, for example, can turn out to have several different meanings. One client may think of independence in terms of the number of times he or she can determine his or her activities for an entire day. Another client may consider independence living on one's own. Still another client might see independence in terms of paying his or her own cost of living. Values need to be specified in observable and measurable terms before they can be truly understood.

In the process of operationalizing values, it may also become clear that what initially appeared to be a single value is, in fact, two or more values. For example, a client may indicate a desire to live in a place that is convenient. When the practitioner explores what the client means by this value, she or he discovers that "convenience" refers both to being close to work and to being close to follow-up treatment. Each of these values may then be defined: *convenience to work* — amount of time it takes to get to work; *convenience to treatment* — amount of time it takes to get to treatment. The check step, then, for knowing when a value has been operationalized involves making sure that it contains only one major element.

Values are important in the decision making process because it is the relative strength of the different values and the resource's comparative ability to satisfy the values that influence which resource is eventually selected. Most community resources, for example, have a cost attached to them. In deciding between them, the presence or absence of cost cannot be the discriminator. However, if it is understood what amounts of cost would be acceptable and what amounts of cost would be unacceptable, it then may be possible to differentiate between alternatives. Similarly, alternative resources may rate differentially across values. One resource may be better on cost but worse on the amount of time the client has to wait for service. Another resource may be worse on cost but provide quicker service. A differentiation cannot be made between alternatives unless the relative importance a client places on cost and speed of service is known. The full operationalization of values permits such precise decision making.

The operationalization of values can take place simultaneously with the identification of values or after the values have been identified. If the client is not familiar with stating values in observable and measurable terms (as most people are not), the joint efforts of the practitioner and client on initial values may translate into the client's ability to independently operationalize values that are identified later. It is important to remember that all the tasks in community service coordination are meant to be cooperative activities between the practitioner and the client.

The skills of operationalizing values include: (1) defining the value as an observable, measurable behavior; (2) scaling the value; and (3) weighting the value.

Defining the Values as an Observable, Measurable Behavior

The first skill in operationalizing a value is to represent the client's value in terms that are observable and measurable — that is, as a behavior. This enables the practitioner and the client to verify their mutual understanding of the client's preference. A basic strategy for specifying the value in behavioral terms is to have the client visualize an activity that represents the preference. Thus, the client who states a preference for independence may visualize doing something that he or she chooses. Another client with the same value may visualize telling his or her parents what he or she thinks or feels about an issue. One client may visualize the value of cost as a person fatigued and drained; another client may visualize cost in terms of spending money to buy something. In any event, the client's picture or visualization of the activity represents the preference.

For example, consider the case of Paul. Paul is a client whose goal is to find "a stable and effective living situation as indicated by being able to live there for at least one year." Paul is a young man who had been hospitalized twice. Although it was not the reason for Paul's last hospitalization, he also had a drinking problem. He had been living with his parents at the time of his last admission, but Paul and the practitioner decided that he should explore an alternative living situation. In the diagnostic plan they developed, they decided that a supervised living experience would be best (e.g., a group home, supervised apartment, or family care program). After the practitioner and Paul had identified several resources that met Paul's goal and for which he is eligible, they attempted to understand Paul's values with respect to the critical areas of cost, availability, accessibility, and acceptability. They next identified other values that seemed important in making this decision. All of these values are defined as a behavior in Table 13.

Notice that the definition of a value also includes a *why* for the value to be measured or quantified. Quantifying the value simply means expressing the value or preference as an amount or as a frequency of occurrence within a specified period of time. The value of independence could be defined as doing what a person wanted to do. The value might be quantified as the number of times in a week that the client was able to do what he or she chose. Similarly, another person

37

might define independence as the activity of telling one's parents what one felt and thought about an issue. The value can then be quantified as a frequency or as a ratio: the ratio of the number of times the person said what he or she thought and felt about an issue to the number of times that issue was discussed. Another way to express the ratio would be as a percentage: the percentage of times the person told his or her parents what he or she thought and felt about an issue. Still a third example might involve cost. A client may represent cost as the activity of spending money. Straightforwardly, this can be quantified as the amount of money paid for a given service.

Table 13. Operationalized Values (Paul)

Values	Operationalization
Cost	Amount of money I will have to pay each month
Availability	Amount of time I will have to wait after discharge period before I can move in
Location	Number of miles to public transportation
Supervision	Accessibility of a Breathalyzer for "hassle-free" monitoring of drinking
Opportunity for making friends	Number of other residents with whom I have something in common (e.g., sports interests)
Privacy	Number of people to a room
Competence	The percentage of self-care tasks (budgeting, cooking, laundering, etc.) I will be allowed to perform

Practice Situations

Consider the following values: freedom, learning, better performance in a student or work role, and increased strength. Take each of these values and try to visualize an activity that represents that particular value for you. Define the value in terms of that activity.

Scaling the Value

The next skill in the operationalizing process is to develop scales that indicate different levels of favorability of a value. Scaling allows for finer discrimination between alternatives that respond favorably to a particular value but to a different degree. For example, two services may each be inexpensive. However, one may cost four dollars per hour and another two dollars per hour. Scaling allows for finer discrimination of the degree to which values or preferences are delivered by different resources.

Once a behavior has been defined in observable and measurable terms, it can be scaled in terms of levels of favorability. Typically, five levels of favorability are scaled. These levels range from level 1 (very unfavorable) to level 5 (very favorable). Each intervening level has the following definition: level 2, unfavorable; level 3, acceptable; and level 4, favorable. Developing favorability scales helps the practitioner and the client to precisely understand each value so that the particular preference can be used to finely discriminate among alternative resources.

To develop favorability scales, the practitioner and the client explore three questions: (1) What quantity of the value would be considered very favorable by the client (level 5)? (2) What quantity of the value would be considered very unfavorable (level 1)? And (3) what quantity of the value would be considered acceptable (level 3)? After these three levels have been identified, the remaining levels of the scale (level 2, unfavorable; and level 4, favorable) can be interpolated.

Turning back now to Jane, from whose case excerpts were previously provided, we can demonstrate the implementation of defining and scaling.

Practitioner: All right, Jane, let's try this scaling once more. Another value you expressed was the speed with which you could obtain the service. Tell me again how you visualize the particular value.

Client: Well, I see myself attending the first session. That's what it means to me.

Practitioner: OK. I guess we can easily define that activity in terms of the amount of time it takes before you can attend that first session. How does that sound?

Client: Sounds fine to me. I've said before that I want to get going soon. I guess the ideal or most favorable situation to me would be to start tomorrow. I guess the worst possible thought is that I will have to wait two or three weeks before I can start acting on what we've identified as a real need of mine. I can live with a week's delay.

Practitioner: Fine. You just identified levels five, one, and three. Let me write that down (see Table 14). Level five would be February twenty-fifth or sooner. Level one would be — let me check the calendar here — March eleventh or later. Level three would be March fourth. OK. How about what would be better than acceptable but not really ideal or very favorable?

Client:	Well, I guess we could just say that what would be good would be after the twenty-fifth and before the fourth. We could do the same thing for level two. Anything after the fourth and before the eleventh would be not as bad as bad could be.
Practitioner:	OK. Fine. Let me write that down. What you are saying is that level four would be having the first session between February twenth-sixth and March third and level two would be having the first session between March fifth and March tenth. I guess this really underlines what you were saying earlier about how anxious you are to get going and how concerned you are that if you aren't able to move fast you're going to lose some of the edge you have built.
Client:	Yeah. I don't want to say I'm scared, but I guess I'm really eager to get started.

The previous excerpt provides one example of scaling a value. It incorporates the first skill of representing the value as an activity as well as the scaling itself. Several other points can be made about the development of scales. First, as indicated in the previous example, the various points on the scale do not have to be made up of a single quantity. Rather, the points can be made up of a range of quantities and values. This is indicated in Table 14. Second, the scale points do not have to be the same size. Again, this is represented in Table 14: levels 5 and 3 are single dates; levels 4 and 2 are intervals. Third, *all points on the scale do not have to be completed.* Five different quantities of a particular preference or value may not make sense from the client's perspective. For some clients, it may just be too difficult or time consuming. At an extreme, there may be only two points. For example, suppose a client absolutely did not want to live in a place that required more than a half-hour to travel to work. However, the client does not care about any commuting time differences of less than a half-hour. The favorability scale in such an instance would designate only two levels. The scales should ultimately reflect the real differences in the value as the client is able to experience that value. To this end, the practitioner will want to help the client understand the rationale for each point in the scale. Table 14 provides an example of levels of favorability scales for all of Jane's values.

Table 14.   Favorability Scales for Values (Jane)

Value: Date of First Session

Levels: (5) February 25 or sooner
(4) February 25 - March 3
(3) March 4
(2) March 5 - 10
(1) March 11 or later

Value: Paying for Service

Levels: (5) No cost
(4) $1 per session
(3) $2 per session
(2) $3 per session
(1) $3 per session

Value: Being Able to *Act* More Successfully

Levels: (5) Teach a skill *and* its application
(4) Teach a skill
(3) Talk and show skills
(2) Talk skills
(1) Don't talk skills or anything

Value: What They Say Fits Who I Am

Levels: (5) Could accurately reflect concern for picking the best resource during my information-seeking contacts
(4)
(3) Provide information freely
(2) Were defensive and hesitant in sharing information
(1) Interpreted my information-seeking as unnecessary or treated it as part of "my problem"

Value: Traveling to Service Location

Levels: (5) Can walk it
(4) One bus away
(3) Two buses away
(2)
(1) Accessible by car only

Value: Openness to Black Clients

Levels: (5) Percentage of black clients and black delivery staff proportional to size of black community
(4) Percentage of black clients proportional to size of black community (only)
(3) Percentage of black delivery staff proportional to size of black community (only)
(2)
(1) Neither percentage of black clients or percentage of staff is proportional to size of black community; *or* no information available

Value: Showing Recognition of My Strengths

Levels: (5) Provide feedback on strengths and deficits based on skills diagnosis
(4)
(3) Use skills diagnosis
(2) Do not diagnose
(1) Use traditional diagnostic methods

Practice Situations

Using your previous practice exercise in defining values, take each of those activities and clearly indicate how you can scale the amount or frequency of the value. Identify the levels of the activity that you would consider most ideal or very favorable, the levels of activity you would consider very unfavorable, and finally, the levels of behavior you would consider acceptable. With these three points defined, turn your attention to filling in the quantities for levels 2 and 4 — unfavorable and favorable respectively. Do this exercise for each of the values you defined in the previous practice exercise.

Weighting the Values

Weighting the values means assigning a relative importance to each value. The fact that values vary in significance needs to be taken into consideration. Assigning weights or numbers that represent the varying significance of values facilitates the decision-making process.

This skill involves ranking the values and assigning weights to values. Values are ranked from most important to least important. Ranking creates a relative scale: that is, although all of the identified values may be important, some values are clearly more important than others.

The practitioner can begin the weighting process by exploring with the client the following questions. *Which value is most important?* The value that best answers this question is placed at the top of the list. The question may then be reversed. *Which value is the least important?* This value is placed at the bottom of the list. The client may then choose to identify which of the values is of average importance to him or her. If such an identification is possible, this value may be placed in the middle of the list. Subsequent to these identifications, the client may then put in order those remaining values that are experienced as relatively more important and place them between the value previously identified as most important and the value previously identified as of average importance. Similarly, the client may order those values that are experienced in the lower half and place them in position between the value previously identified as of average importance and the value previously identified as least important.

One way to facilitate the ranking process may be to write each value on separate sheets of paper or index cards. The client may then sort through the cards and select the most important value, the least important value, and the value of average importance. The remaining cards can be divided into those that are of more than average importance and those that are of less than average importance. Indeed, the entire task can be given to some clients as a homework assignment. Clients who have a low level of functioning may need to be guided through the ranking process step by step.

Once the values have been ranked according to importance, the next step is to assign corresponding weights or numbers. The weighting process uses the following scale: 10 = most important; 5 = average importance; and 1 = least important. The weights or numbers 2 through 4 are used for less important values, and the numbers 6 through 9 are used for relatively more important values. If more than ten values have been identified by a client, it is recommended that the scale be extended in range from, perhaps, 20 to 1. Creating an adequate spread to the weights is important for the purpose of making the difference between alternatives clear.

If others are involved in the client's rehabilitation, the practitioner may want to include them in the process of weighting values, as well as in the process of identifying and operationalizing values. If agreement on a weight cannot be reached through discussion, the simplest way to resolve different perspectives on the relative importance of values is to take an average of the weights each individual assigned the particular value. Thus, for example, if two parents were working with a practitioner to decide the best type of place for their child to live and one of the parents gave the value of "expense" a weight of 9 while the other parent weighted it 5, a compromise weight would be 7.

Throughout the value definition, scaling, and weighting process, the practitioner is guided by the principle of trying to *maximize the client's involvement* in the value operationalization process. Thus, a process that gets too detailed or too complex for the client will tend to reduce client involvement. If the practitioner senses that this is occurring, he or she can simplify the process. If necessary, the practitioner can define the values for the client, based on the client's exploration. Values do not have to be systematically scaled; the practitioner can just elicit from the client what is acceptable and what is not. The weighting process can be simplified so that the client merely identifies two groups of values: (1) values that are "important," and (2) values that are "really important." The critical purpose of the value operationalization process is to gain a perspective of the client's relevant values and preferences that is understandable to both *the client and the practitioner*. It is only when the client understands the value operationalization process that the client can become maximally involved in choosing the best available community resource — based on the client's own unique value system.

Practice Situations

An example of a completed list of weighted values is provided in Table 15. Recorded in this table are the values identified for the client Jane. As a practice exercise, weight the values you previously identified for yourself. Which of these values would you rank as most important? Which would you place as least important? Complete the remaining steps of weighting values.

Table 15. Weighted Values (Jane)

Value	Weight
Cost	5
Speed of service entry	10
Location	1
Openness to black clients	8
Skills orientation	9
Emphasis on strengths	7
Ability to relate to me as I am	6

UNDERSTANDING THE CLIENT'S VALUES AND PREFERENCES: A SUMMARY

Goal: To minimize the possiblity of failure in community service co-ordination by ensuring that the selected resource will be experienced by the client as worthwhile and acceptable

1. Orient the client to the exploration of values.

2. Elicit the client's preferences for cost, availability, accessibility, and acceptability.

3. Identify other client preferences.

4. Operationalize the client's values and preferences. (a) Define the value as an observable, measurable behavior. (b) Scale the value. (c) Weight the value.

RESEARCHING THE POTENTIAL COMMUNITY RESOURCE ALTERNATIVES

At this stage in the community resource selection process, the practitioner and the client have selected potential community resource alternatives and operationalized those client values that will be critical in identifying the best of the available resources.

The next major skill in choosing the appropriate community resource is to research the potential alternatives with respect to how well they might be able to satisfy the client's values. The research process involves gathering the specific information necessary to assess the potential of each alternative resource to satisfy the values of the client. For example, to assist a client to achieve the goal of having people within his or her living environment who can teach the skills of daily living, practitioner and client might be considering the alternatives of a family-care placement, a halfway house, or a supervised apartment supplemented by a five-day-per-week day-care program. In investigating the value of expense, the client or practitioner will investigate the cost of each of these alternatives: the cost of the halfway house program per month, the cost of the supervised apartment program supplemented by the day-care program per month, and the cost of family-care placement per month. This research would provide the essential information necessary to evaluate each of the three alternatives on the value dimension of expense.

Researching potential alternatives involves two subskills: planning the research effort, and implementing the research plan.

PLANNING THE RESEARCH EFFORT

The development of a research plan involves identifying *what* will be researched, *who* will do the research, the *source* of information, how and when the information will be obtained, and how the information will be recorded. Identification of what will be researched and who will do the research labels the individual who will be responsible for seeking the information needed and the specific information he or she will seek.

Essentially, any party involved in the rehabilitation process, whether it be the client, the practitioner, or a third party participating with the consent of the client, may assume the responsibility for pursuing information concerning potential alternatives. In general, the more the client can do on his or her own behalf, the more benefits he or she experiences. Further, the act of participation tends to support greater investment in the ultimate decision that is made.

In determining what will be researched, the practitioner and the client can draw specific guidance from their previous work in developing and operationalizing the client's values and preferences. The operationalized values of the client represent the specific focuses for information gathering, since it is these values against which each potential alternative is to be assessed. Table 16 provides an example of the use of operationalized values to formulate questions for the research effort. The values and questions contained in Table 16 are for the client Jane. As can be seen, the translation of questions from values is straightforward and simple. Thus, the value of speed of service entry, which was operationalized as the date of the first session, translates into the question: What would be the earliest date that Jane could begin to receive services?

As can also be seen from the table, each value may generate more than one question. Thus, openness to black clients was operationalized as involving the concept of both the ratio of blacks served to blacks in the community and the ratio of blacks on staff to blacks in the community. Thus, multiple questions would be required in order to obtain enough information to select a potential resource on this particular value.

Table 16.   Sample Questions for Operationalized Values (Jane)

Operationalized Value	Question(s)
Date of first session Speed of service entry:	What would be the earliest date that Jane could begin to receive services?
Traveling to service location Location:	Where is the specific program Jane would receive located? What public transportation can be used to get to the site?
Paying for service Cost:	What is the fee for service? What accommodation is made for people who are unable to pay?
Openness to black clients	What proportion of all clients served are black? What is the ratio of blacks served to blacks in the community? What percentage of the *delivery* staff is black? What steps are taken to attract and retain black clients?
Being able to act more successfully Skills orientation:	What is the orientation of the service? What does it hope to do for clients? What steps are included to assist clients to *act* more effectively?
Showing recognition of my strengths Emphasis on strengths:	What is included in the assessment process? What specific feedback is given to the client about the assessment? How are the results of assessment used in service delivery?
What they say fits who I am Ability to relate to me as I am:	How accurately has the service responded to my questions? How accurately has the service responded to where I am coming from in asking the questions? What is the feedback of clients on how effectively they were understood?

Once it is understood what questions need to be answered and who will be seeking the information, it is then necessary to identify from what source the information is to be obtained. There are two sources of information: people and written material. People sources include persons who are employed by the resource as well as individuals who are connected to the resource but not directly employed by it.

Included in this latter group would be individuals who volunteer in an agency or program, persons who may be on the governing board, persons who may be in evaluation and monitoring roles, and persons who may have previously worked at a facility. Written materials include brochures and pamphlets published by the resource, referral materials distributed by the resource, listings of the resource in centralized community service directories, and information obtained by a practitioner as a result of previous experience with the resource.

The source for obtaining any particular information is selected on the basis of its accessibility and the likelihood of its having the information needed. Naturally, materials in hand represent the most accessible source. Individuals who could be readily contacted by phone or seen face to face represent another fairly accessible resource. However, in some instances, the type of information needed will require reaching for possibly less accessible resources. This may be the case with reference to information about the efficacy of a program, its precise nature, and its sensitivity to minorities. Obtaining this type of information may require contacting former clients, checking with colleagues who have used the resource previously, and talking to minority groups within the community. In the case of Jane, for example, her concern about the resource's openness to serving blacks might require that she contact the local Urban League to identify whether any complaints have been made concerning the resource and obtain an annual report to see what percentage of the clients served in the last calendar year were black, or if, indeed, the agency is even sensitive enough to monitor its relative services to minorities in the community.

Essentially, the remaining steps of researching the potential alternatives continue the effort at being organized and systematic. The more planned the researching of alternatives is, the more likely it is to be completed — and completed in a manner that facilitates decision making. The planning effort is even more important when the client, or an involved significant other, is investigating the resource in question. In these instances, the planning works to support their successful involvement.

Identifying the *how* and *when* of researching simply means specifying the method by which the information will be obtained and when it will be obtained. A decision must also be made about the way in which the obtained information will be recorded and brought back into the rehabilitation setting.

IMPLEMENTING THE RESEARCH PLAN

The implementation of the research plan is simple when a clear plan has been developed. As an example, Jane was able to research her potential alternatives and obtain the information provided in Table 17. The decision to involve Jane in gathering the information was a good one. Jane was able to get a "feeling" for the potential alternatives and to gather information on her resource's "ability to relate to me as I am" value.

Table 17. Information Obtained in Researching Potential Alternatives (Jane)

Value	Community Mental Health Center	Community College	Women's Task Force
Cost	Billed cost: $28.65 per session; expected payment approximately $1 per session. Remainder billed to Title XX	Billed cost: averages $15 per class; no direct payment required since Vocational Rehabilitation Commission will subsidize	Billed cost: $0 per session; program subsidized by grant
Speed of service entry	February 28	June 20	March 2
Location	One bus ride	Two buses	One bus ride
Openness to black clients	Information not immediately available	Percentage of black students does not parallel percentage of blacks in community; percentage of blacks on staff is very low	Percentage of black clients parallels percentage of blacks in community; percentage of black staff is low
Skills orientation	Psychodynamically oriented; insight; use of drugs	Ideal oriented; study concepts and principles	Behaviorally oriented; skills identified and demonstrations used
Emphasis on strengths	*APA*, DSM II classification system	Evaluation of high school performance for entrance	No formal assessment made
Ability to relate to me as I am	Defensive on telephone about all the questions being asked; said that some information was not available; wanted to know why information was sought	Offered information; said they were eager to let people know about themselves	Mixed; at first seemed suspicious of questions; then, after exploration, shared information readily

Practice Situations

As a practice exercise, review the values you previously identified for yourself. Using the values as a guide, generate the specific questions you would need to ask the particular resource in order to discover the information required to assess where that resource stands in relation to your particular concern.

Select three community resources to research as alternatives. In selecting the resources, choose those you are likely to use in future community service coordination efforts. Prepare to research the questions you have identified by first determining the best source for the information and then planning how and when you will gain access to the source. Complete the researching process and record the information you have obtained in a format similar to Table 17.

RESEARCHING THE POTENTIAL COMMUNITY RESOURCE ALTERNATIVES: A SUMMARY

Goal: To gather the information that is necessary to assess the ability of each of the potential resource alternatives to meet the client's values and preferences

1. Identify what information is needed (e.g., the questions to be answered) and who will obtain the information.
2. Identify the source of the information.
3. Identify how and when the information will be obtained and recorded.
4. Obtain and record the information.

CHOOSING THE APPROPRIATE COMMUNITY RESOURCE

The final major skill in selecting the appropriate community resource is to actually choose the preferred resource. The decision-making process integrates the perspective of the client and the information about each resource alternative into a final determination of who may best serve the client's needs. Thus, the final step of selecting a resource can be implemented only when the client's perspective has been fully operationalized and each community resource alternative fully understood.

Choosing the appropriate community resource involves four subskills: (1) assessing the resource's conformity to the client's preferences; (2) computing the resource's desirability; (3) identifying the most desirable resource; and (4) recycling the decision-making efforts to ensure the development of an adequate alternative. *Assessing the resource's conformity to client preferences* means knowing where each

49

potential community resource stands in relation to the client's values. *Computing the resource's desirability* means calculating the extent to which each resource meets the client's preference. *Identifying the most desirable community resource* means labeling the resource that minimally meets the client's values and preferences. *Recycling the decision-making efforts* means modifying existing alternatives to more fully meet the client's needs and preferences.

There are instances, of course, when the client and the practitioner will not go through the level of systematization in choosing the preferred resource. This is usually due to one of two reasons: (1) based on the information collected during the researching of alternatives, one alternative can be seen to be clearly superior in its ability to satisfy the client's values, or (2) the level of detail needed to most comprehensively and systematically decide on a resource hinders rather than facilitates client involvement.

In the first instance, the data obtained from researching the resources will seem to overwhelmingly indicate the desirability of one resource. A look at the information collected will show one resource to be outstanding in its ability to satisfy most of the client's important values. The decision is clear. All that remains is for the practitioner to check to see if there is any way to make the resource area more satisfying to the client.

In the second instance, the practitioner will sense that the level of detail and/or the use of numbers in the decision-making process might overwhelm the client. This may be the same type of client who needed the value operationalization process simplified. In such situations, the practitioner might simply wish to do a "yes-no" assessment of whether or not a resource satisfies each of the client values. The preferred resource would simply be the resource with the greatest number of "yes" assessments for the client's most important values. The key to meaningful decision making is to get the client to indicate, based on the most accurate resource information available, whether or not a resource will satisfy each of the client's values. *The preferred resource is that resource which conforms most closely to the client's value system.* How systematic one becomes in making this assessment is a function of what level of systematization will be helpful to the client. The decision-making process outlined in the next several pages is quite systematic. Once the practitioner has mastered the decision-making skills at this level of detail, he or she will also be able to simplify the decision-making process when the client's need or situation so dictates.

ASSESSING THE RESOURCE'S CONFORMITY TO THE CLIENT'S PREFERENCES

The skill of assessing the resource's conformity to the client's preferences involves assigning each resource a rating for each of the client's values, based on the favorability scales developed and the research completed on each particular resource. The process of assessing a resource is accomplished by (1) reviewing the information about the resource in relation to each client value and (2) identifying what level of favorability the resource achieves for the particular value.

An example of assessing a resource's conformity to client preferences is provided in Table 18. Here, the values developed and scaled for the client Jane (Table 14) have been used to evaluate the information obtained for the Community Mental Health Center. A favorability score is reported for each value. Thus, for the first value, cost, a review of the information provided in Table 17 indicates that the Community Mental Health Center would charge approximately one dollar per session. Given Jane's scaling of the value cost, the charge of one dollar per session results in a favorability score of 4. Hence, the number 4 would be placed in the column under Community Mental Health Center opposite the value of cost (Table 18). Similarly, the Community Mental Health Center was able to provide an initial-session date of February 28. Again, review of Jane's favorability scale for speed of service entry indicates that the date of service would achieve a favorability score of 4. Using a similar process, the remaining assessment of the Community Mental Health Center, relative to each value, was completed. The results indicated that the Community Mental Health Center, as a resource alternative, achieved a favorability score of 4 on "location," 1 on "openness to black clients," 1 on "skills orientation," 1 on "emphasis on strengths," and 2 on "ability to relate to me as I am."

Table 18.   Partially Completed Assessment of
Resource Conformity to Client Preferences (Jane)

Value	Community Mental Health Center	Community College	Women's Task Force
Cost	4		
Speed of service entry	4		
Location	4		
Openness to black clients	1		
Skills orientation	1		
Emphasis on strengths	1		
Ability to relate to me as I am	2		

Practice Situations

As a practice exercise, complete the assessment of the community resource alternatives: Community College and Women's Task Force. Use the procedures previously described. The information required is provided in Tables 14 and 17. Once you have completed the exercise, check your answers against those provided in Table 19.

Table 19. Completed Assessment of Resource
            Conformity to Client Preferences (Jane)

Value	Community Mental Health Center	Community College	Women's Task Force
Cost	4	5	5
Speed of service entry	4	1	4
Location	4	3	4
Openness to black clients	1	1	4
Skills orientation	1	1	4
Emphasis on strengths	1	1	2
Ability to relate to me as I am	2	3	2

COMPUTING THE RESOURCE'S DESIRABILITY

Computing the resource alternative's desirability means calculating the extent to which the resource meets the client's concerns. The computation brings together two pieces of information that reflect on the client's concerns: the favorability scale (defining the levels of value fulfillment) and the weight (defining the importance of the value). The combined data are summarized over all values for each resource alternative. Hence, each resource alternative receives a desirability score that reflects the weighted degree to which it succeeds in meeting the requirements of each value.

Table 20 provides an example of computing a resource's desirability — in this case, for the Community Mental Health Center alternative. As can be seen, *the favorability scores are multiplied by the weight* and *the results are summed* to complete the computation of the desirability score. The Community Mental Health Center alternative achieves a desirability score of 100.

Table 20. Sample Computation of Resource Desirability (Jane)

Value	Weight	Community Mental Health Center
Cost	5	× 4 = 20
Speed of service entry	10	× 4 = 40
Location	1	× 4 = 4
Openness to black clients	8	× 1 = 8
Skills orientation	9	× 1 = 9
Emphasis on strengths	7	× 1 = 7
Ability to relate to me as I am	6	× 2 = 12
Desirability score		100

Practice Situations

As a practice exercise, complete the computations for the Community College and the Women's Task Force. After you complete the task, check your answers, using the information provided in Table 21.

Table 21. Completed Computation of Resource Desirability (Jane)

Value	Weight	Community Mental Health Center	Community College	Women's Task Force
Cost	5	× 4 = 20	× 5 = 25	× 5 = 25
Speed of service entry	10	× 4 = 40	× 1 = 10	× 4 = 40
Location	1	× 4 = 4	× 3 = 3	× 4 = 4
Openness to black clients	8	× 1 = 8	× 1 = 8	× 4 = 32
Skills orientation	9	× 1 = 9	× 1 = 9	× 3 = 27
Emphasis on strengths	7	× 1 = 7	× 1 = 7	× 2 = 14
Ability to relate to me as I am	6	× 2 = 12	× 3 = 18	× 2 = 12
Desirability score		100	80	154

IDENTIFYING THE MOST DESIRABLE RESOURCE

At this point the practitioner can identify the resource that would be most satisfying and acceptable to the client. Determining the most desirable resource involves computing the average weighted desirability score achieved by each alternative, determining whether any alternative achieves at least an acceptable average weighted level of desirability, that is, an average of 3.0, and, finally, labeling the alternative that scores highest above the acceptable level of desirability.

The subskills involved in identifying the most appropriate resource are: (1) determining the sum of the weights; (2) dividing the desirability score achieved by each alternative by the sum of the weights; (3) identifying which, if any, resource achieves at least an acceptable average weighted desirability score; and (4) identifying which scores highest above that level.

Table 21 provides a full computation of the desirability scores in the case of Jane's resource alternatives. Also listed in the table are the weights for each of the values identified by Jane and her practitioner. First, to identify the most appropriate resource, the sum of the weights is obtained. In this instance, the sum equals 46 (5 + 10 + 1 + 8 + 9 + 7 + 6 = 46). To compute the average weighted favorability score for the Community Mental Health Center alternative, the desirability score of the Community Mental Health Center (100) is divided by the sum of the weights (46). The resulting dividend is 2.17 (100 : 46 = 2.17). When the process is completed for each of the remaining resource alternatives, the results are: Community College, 1.74 (80 : 46 = 1.74); Women's Task Force, 3.35 (154 : 46 = 3.35). Table 22 presents the results of these calculations. As can be seen, the Women's Task Force offers a program that achieves at least an acceptable level of average weighted favorability (3.00 = acceptable level). Hence, the community resource identified as most appropriate is the Women's Task Force.

Table 22. Computation of the Resource's Average Weighted Desirability (Jane)

Values	Weight	Community Mental Health Center	Community College	Women's Task Force
Cost	5	× 4 = 20	× 5 = 25	× 5 = 25
Speed of service entry	10	× 4 = 40	× 1 = 10	× 4 = 40
Location	1	× 4 = 4	× 3 = 3	× 4 = 4
Openness to black clients	8	× 1 = 8	× 1 = 8	× 4 = 32
Skills orientation	9	× 1 = 9	× 1 = 9	× 3 = 27
Emphasis on strengths	7	× 1 = 7	× 1 = 7	× 2 = 14
Ability to relate to me as I am	6	× 2 = 12	× 3 = 18	× 2 = 12
Desirability score		100	80	154
Average weighted desirability		2.17	1.74	3.35

Practice Situations

Table 23 provides a sample format for computing the desirability of three alternative sources for emergency fuel allocations. The three alternatives are being considered by Mrs. King as ways of resolving her heating problem. In the decision-making matrix are listed Mrs. King's values, the weights, and the scores achieved by each alternative. Using a format similar to Table 22, compute for each alternative the average weighted desirability score, and identify which alternative is the most appropriate resource for her to use. After you have completed the exercise, you can check the accuracy of your answers with the information provided in Table 24.

Table 23. Demonstrating Choosing the Most Desirable Alternative (Mrs. Jane King)

Values	Weight	Alternative Community Resources		
		Community Action Corporation	Council of Churches	Mrs. King's Children
Outcome	(10)	4 ___	4 ___	5 ___
Speed	(7)	4 ___	4 ___	5 ___
Location	(5)	3 ___	2 ___	4 ___
Privacy	(3)	3 ___	3 ___	4 ___
Self-sufficiency	(9)	4 ___	4 ___	1 ___
Desirability score				
Average weighted desirability				

Table 24. Computations for Choosing the Most Desirable Alternative (Mrs. King)

Value	Weight	Community Action Commission		Council of Churches		Children	
Outcome	10	4	40	4	40	5	50
Speed	7	4	28	4	28	5	35
Location	5	3	15	2	10	4	20
Privacy	3	3	9	3	9	4	12
Self-sufficiency	9	4	36	4	36	1	9
Desirability score		128		123		126	
Average weighted desirability		3.76		3.61		3.71	

RECYCLING THE DECISION-MAKING EFFORTS

In some instance, no resource will achieve an average weighted desirability score of 3.0 or higher. This means that no community resource alternative achieved a generally acceptable level of satisfaction for the client's identified values. If this occurs, there are three possible ways to develop a viable alternative for the client: (1) modifying an alternative resource already evaluated in the decision-making matrix; (2) reconsidering alternative resources; and (3) developing new resource alternatives.

Modifying an Alternative Resource

The first step in attempting to develop a viable alternative is to determine if one of the existing resources can be improved. This may be accomplished by working with a resource and/or the client to overcome the resource's potential deficits.

The process by which an alternative can be improved to increase its favorability for the client can be systematically described in four steps, as illustrated in the case of John. John is a client whose goal is to "find an educational program that he can stay with." He is a young man who has been hospitalized repeatedly. Although it was not the reason for the most recent admission, he had a drug problem in the past (use of LSD). He had been living in the school dormitory prior to his last admission but is currently living with his sister and her family. Over the past eight years, John has been enrolled at four universities, has majored in sociology, and has completed the equivalent of one year's credits. John and his practitioner decided that a local educational program that would allow him to continue his present living situation would be best. They brainstormed the alternatives; developed, scaled, and weighted the values; researched the alternatives; and completed a decision-making matrix. Tables 25 and 26 present John's favorability scales, weights, and decision-making matrix. Although the trade or vocational school alternative emerges as slightly better than the other alternatives, it does not prove to be a truly acceptable alternative for John. The average weighted favorability score is less than 3.00.

Table 25. Favorability Scales and Weights (John)

Value	Weight	Level	Scale
Degree offered	9	5	Bachelor's degree or higher
		4	
		3	Two-year degree (e.g., associate)
		2	
		1	No degree
Eligibility	10	5	Grade-point-average of 2.50 or less
		4	
		3	
		2	
		1	Grade-point-average of 2.51 or more
Time	8	5	One to two years
		4	
		3	Two to four years
		2	
		1	More than four years
Potential friends	1	5	75 to 100 percent
		4	61 to 74 percent
		3	49 to 60 percent
		2	25 to 48 percent
		1	Less than 24 percent
Supervision	4	5	Advisor available upon demand
		4	
		3	Advisor available by appointment
		2	
		1	No advisor available
Instructors	5	5	Weekly office hours, plus ten minutes after class
		4	
		3	Weekly office hours
		2	
		1	No interaction time built in
Flexibility in requirements	7	5	Requirements negotiable
		4	
		3	Some alternatives for each requirement
		2	
		1	Rigid program requirements
Course compatibility	8	5	80–100 percent deal with interests
		4	
		3	50–70 percent deal with interests
		2	
		1	Less than 50 percent deal with interests
Internships	6	5	51–75 percent of course work hours
		4	
		3	25–50 percent of course work hours
		2	
		1	Less than 25 percent of course work hours

Table 26. Decision-Making Matrix (John)

Value	Weight	Local University Favorability Level	Score	Local Junior College Favorability Level	Score	Trade or Vocational School Favorability Level	Score	Continuing Education Favorability Level	Score
Degree offered	9	5	45	3	27	2	18	1	9
Eligibility	10	1	10	1	10	5	50	5	50
Time	8	3	24	5	40	5	40	5	40
Potential friends	1	2	2	1	1	1	1	3	3
Supervision	4	3	12	3	12	3	12	1	4
Instructors	5	5	25	5	25	3	15	1	5
Flexibility in requirements	7	1	7	3	21	1	7	5	35
Course compatibility	8	3	24	3	24	1	8	1	8
Internships	6	1	6	1	6	5	30	1	6
Desirability score			155		166		171		160

Highest alternative score   = 171

$$\frac{171 \text{ (Highest alternative score)}}{58 \text{ (sum of weights)}} = 2.94 \text{ (average weighted desirability)}$$

The first step in attempting to improve the existing alternatives is to list the weak areas of each. For each alternative, those values for which the alternative resource scored less than level 3 ("acceptable") would be listed. For example, the areas in which John's highest-scoring alternative, trade or vocational school, fell short of acceptability were "degree offered," "potential friends," "flexibility in requirements," and "course compatibility." For each deficit value, it was then helpful for the practitioner and John to explore the change that would be necessary to make the resource score at least acceptable (level 3). For example, for the trade or vocational school alternative to reach an acceptable score on the value of the type of degree offered, it would have to offer at least a two-year degree.

The second step is to consider whether the educational program, if it were willing, could change in order to become an acceptable alternative. The practitioner and John developed a brief "yes" or "no" checklist to indicate the possibility of each resource modifying its program. This step serves as a "reality" check on the probability of the resource changing to fit the client's needs. Although an educational resource might accept a student who did not meet eligibility requirements, it would be unlikely that the resource could offer a degree for a nondegree program. In order to complete this step, the practitioner and client discuss and agree on what changes are needed and the likelihood of these specific changes being made. For example, when discussing ways to make the courses offered by the trade or vocational school more compatible with John's interests. John and the practitioner determined that the specific change of adding sociology courses was impossible.

The third step is to write a description of each resource, including the realistic changes (i.e., those changes checked "yes"). The description includes the name of the resource, what changes are necessary, who can provide the change, and how the change would be made. To complete this step, the practitioner and/or the client might need to reuse the previously described research skills to obtain the information necessary to write a full description of the modified resource. Table 27 shows the weak areas, the reality check, and the development of descriptive change statements for each of John's resource alternatives.

The last step is to evaluate the modified resource alternative. The procedures involved are the same as those used in the initial decision-making process. Table 28 presents the revised decision-making matrix that was used to evaluate the modified alternatives developed for John and to choose the preferred modified resource. The improved alternative of the local university emerges as the preferred educational resource for John. The average weighted desirability score indicates that the local university is generally favorable in terms of meeting all the values developed by John and his practitioner.

Table 27. Development of Modified Resource Alternatives (John)

Alternatives	Weak Areas (deficit values)	Reality Check		Descriptive Change Statements
		Yes	No	
Trade or vocational school	1. Degree offered		X	No change possible.
	2. Potential friends		X	
	3. Flexibility in requirements		X	
	4. Course compatibility		X	
Continuing education	1. Degree offered		X	The director agrees to work with instructors to offer John interaction time, provide advice, and help develop internship opportunities.
	2. Supervision	X		
	3. Instructors	X		
	4. Course compatibility	X		
	5. Internships		X	
Local junior college	1. Eligibility	X		The Admissions director agrees to lower eligibility requirements for John; the curriculum dean would participate in negotiations for internships.
	2. Potential friends		X	
	3. Internships	X		
Local university	1. Eligibility	X		The Admissions director agrees to reduce eligibility requirements; and the curriculum dean would negotiate requirement alternatives and internships.
	2. Time		X	
	3. Flexibility in requirements	X		
	4. Internships	X		

Table 28. Revised Decision-Making Matrix (John)

Value	Weight	Modified University Favorability		Modified Junior College Favorability		Continuing Education Favorability	
		Level	Score	Level	Score	Level	Score
Degree offered	9	5	45	3	27	1	9
Eligibility	10	5	50	5	50	5	50
Time	8	3	24	5	40	5	40
Potential friends	1	3	3	1	1	3	3
Supervision	4	3	12	3	12	3	12
Instructors	5	5	25	5	25	5	25
Flexibility in requirements	7	3	21	3	21	5	35
Course compatibility	8	3	24	3	24	1	8
Internships	6	3	18	3	18	3	18
Desirability score			222		218		200
Average weighted desirability			3.83		3.77		3.44

Practice Situations

As a practice exercise, work with Katherine, a thirty-year-old woman who was released from the hospital last year. Katherine's practitioner is concerned about which employment agency to use to help Katherine locate appropriate employment. Tables 29 and 30 contain Katherine's favorability scales, weights for values, and decision-making matrix. As shown in the matrix (Table 30), the highest-scoring alternative, C.E.T.A., does not check out as a highly favorable choice for Katherine (average weighted favorability score is only 2.91). Develop modified alternatives for Katherine by listing the weak areas for each resource alternative, estimating the reality of the resource change, and writing a descriptive change statement for each alternative, using a format similar to Table 27.

Using Table 28 as a guideline, evaluate the modified alternatives developed for Katherine.

Reconsidering Alternative Resources

If a viable alternative cannot be developed through modification, the next step is to return to the brainstorming process of identifying alternatives and check whether a potential alternative might have been omitted from the initial list of available community resources. The practitioner will want to make additional contacts and undertake research to uncover any possibility previously missed.

Additional resource alternatives uncovered during this renewed brainstorming effort can be evaluated using the values, weights, and desirability scales already developed. The outcome desired is once again the identification of a preferred alternative that achieves an average weighted desirability score of 3.00.

Table 29. Favorability Scales and Weights (Katherine)

Value	Weight	Level	Scale
Fee	7	5	No fee
		4	
		3	Sliding scale according to income
		2	
		1	Standard fee
Type of clients	8	5	Unemployed psychiatric rehabil-itation clients
		4	
		3	Unemployed clients (one year or more)
		2	
		1	Other
Placement time	10	5	Under three months
		4	Three to four months
		3	Five to seven months
		2	Eight to nine months
		1	Ten months or more
Counselor contact	6	5	More than once a week
		4	
		3	Scheduled weekly meetings
		2	
		1	Less than once a week
Potential client contact	1	5	Group sessions
		4	
		3	
		2	
		1	Individual sessions
Counselor-client relationship	7	5	Responds to client
		4	
		3	Pays attention to client
		2	
		1	Does not pay attention to client
Job placement training	9	5	Offered
		4	
		3	
		2	
		1	Not offered
Sharing of job	5	5	All job openings shared
		4	
		3	Selective job openings shared
		2	
		1	Job openings not shared
Job placement materials	3	5	Library and selection help available
		4	Complete library available
		3	Some materials available
		2	Limited materials available
		1	No library

Table 30. Decision-Making Matrix (Katherine)

Value	Weight	State Bureau of Employment Services		C.E.T.A.		Private Employment Agency	
		Favorability Level	Score	Favorability Level	Score	Favorability Level	Score
Fee	7	5	35	5	35	1	7
Type of clients	8	3	24	3	24	1	8
Placement time	10	1	10	3	30	4	40
Counselor contact	6	1	6	3	18	3	18
Potential client contacts	1	1	1	5	5	1	1
Counselor-client relationship	7	1	7	1	7	3	21
Job placement training	9	1	9	1	9	1	9
Sharing of job openings	5	5	25	5	25	3	15
Job placement materials	3	2	6	3	9	3	9
Desirability score			123		162		128
Average weighted desirability			2.19		2.91		2.28

Developing New Resources

When the alternatives evaluated during the decision-making process are not acceptable and cannot be modified, and when additional alternatives cannot be identified through renewed brainstorming efforts, the practitioner faces the prospect of developing an entirely new resource alternative. The development of a new resource is generally a very large task that goes beyond the scope of authority of the practitioner. Furthermore, new resources are rarely developed in response to the needs of a single client. Nevertheless, it is possible for a practitioner to contribute to the effort of developing new resources within the community that, although perhaps not initiated soon enough to be of help to a present client, can be of help to future clients and other community residents.

The absence of a viable community resource for a particular client indicates, by definition, a lack in available community resources. The practitioner will want to ensure that this lack is filled with an appropriate resource. The practitioner's contribution to this process is his or her understanding of the nature of the resource needed, as developed during the decision-making process. To initiate the process of developing a new resource, the practitioner can contact those community groups responsible for ensuring that adequate community resources exist, institutions that fund resources, and relevant advocacy groups whose mission it is to ensure that responsible agents act to provide for community needs.

The practitioner can begin by using the results of the decision-making matrix to describe exactly the kind of resource that is missing from the community. This can be done by using the most favorable level (level 5) of the values used to evaluate the initial alternatives. For example, if, for John, the most favorable (level 5) degree offered is a bachelor's degree or higher, then one criterion for the new resource is that a bachelor's or higher degree can be obtained from the educational program. Table 31 presents a detailed description of the characteristics that the educational program most desirable for John must meet. Notice that the characteristics are listed in order of importance, based on the weighting of the values.

Table 31. Characteristics of the Preferred Resource (John)

---

1. Acceptance of students with grade-point-averages of less than 2.5

2. Offering of at least a bachelor's degree for completion of program

3. Eighty percent of courses dealing with John's interests (sociology, helping, psychology, social issues, philosophy)

4. Completion of the program to take no more than two years

5. Program requirements negotiable with individual student

6. At least half of the school time spent in student internships

7. At least weekly meetings and brief informal opportunities to talk with instructors

8. Student advisor available to students on demand or when needed

9. At least three-quarters of students in late twenties, returning to school, interested in social issues

---

Next, the practitioner can identify responsible agents for ensuring the adequacy of the human service system. If the problem is in the educational area, the practitioner will want to identify the local authority responsible for ensuring that the community has an adequate educational system. If the problem is in the area of mental health services, the practitioner will want to identify who is responsible for ensuring that adequate mental health services are provided to the community. One way to identify who is responsible in the various sectors would be to review the agencies previously identified as sources of community resource listings. Again, these listings are frequently developed by those agencies responsible for the existence of adequate resources in a human service area. Similarly, it would be worthwhile to identify funding sources for the particular area in which the lack of resources has been identified. Finally, identifying appropriate advocacy groups would complete the development of awareness of who needs to know about the lack of available community resources.

Before initiating contact, however, the practitioner will want to consult with his or her supervisor. A supervisor may already have contact with one of these organizations and may be a liaison with the organization. In this instance, the information developed by the practitioner concerning the lack in resources would be provided to the supervisor for transmission to the appropriate people. If such a liaison

67

person does not exist within the organization, then the process of communicating the discovered lack in available resources can be codetermined with a supervisor. The simplest way would be to draft a letter introducing the lack in service, utilizing the detailed description of the characteristics of the needed service (e.g., Table 31), and providing an estimate of the type of client who would require the resource.

Practice Situations

As a practice exercise, assume that you are unable to modify any of Katherine's alternatives so that they become a preferred resource. Describe the criteria an employment agency must meet to be chosen for Katherine. Next, identify what authorities are responsible for ensuring the adequacy of community resources in the employment area. Since Katherine may qualify as a chronically ill client, given her history of previous psychiatric hospitalizations, consider the possibility of multiple responsible authorities. List the responsible authorities you identified. Identify as well the funding sources that support programs in the area of employment, and programs that provide service for the posthospitalized client.

CHOOSING THE APPROPRIATE COMMUNITY RESOURCE: A SUMMARY

Goal: To select the community resource that will meet the needs of the client in a manner responsive to the client's values and concerns

1. Assess the resource's conformity to the client's preferences.(a) Review the information about the resource in relation to each client value. (b) Identify the level of favorability the resource achieves for each client value.

2. Compute the resource's desirability by multiplying the value weights by the favorability scores and adding the products to determine the total for each resource.

3. Identify the most appropriate resource: (a) determine the sum of the weights; (b) divide the resource's desirability score by the sum of the weights; (c) identify which resource achieves at least an acceptable average weighted desirability score and scores the highest above that level.

4. Recycle decision making: (a) modify an alternative resource previously evaluated; (b) reconsider new alternatives; (c) develop new alternative resources.

SELECTING THE APPROPRIATE COMMUNITY RESOURCE: A SKILLED APPROACH

Wes was determined to stay off drugs, but Shari, Wes's counselor, knew full well that determination alone would not be enough. She had seen too many young people make what they felt was a total, absolute commitment, only to weaken in a matter of a few short weeks when things got tougher than they had anticipated.

"You don't need to be in the hospital," she told Wes. "What would probably be best is a group living facility where you can get the kind of support you need to stay drug-free."

Wes agreed with this. As it turned out, he was also familiar in a very limited way with one particular facility near his family's home. "A place called Westward House, something like that," he said. "I remember a buddy of mine had an older brother who spent time there."

"Yes, I've heard of that one," Shari told him. "I think the name is Westwood House. It might be a good place, too. But I think it's probably too early to just pick a facility right now. There are a lot of things we need to know in order to choose just the right house for you."

"What kind of things?" Wes wanted to know.

"Oh — like how many people are there, for example. Remember, you said you didn't like being crowded wherever you lived, so we wouldn't want to pick a place where everyone lived dormitory-style."

"Yeah, that makes good sense," Wes admitted. "Huh, I never would have thought to check that out."

"There are other considerations, too," Shari told him, "like whether the people are your age or younger, whether the types of drug problems being treated are like yours or of a different kind entirely; what kinds of activities go on, what the supervision is like — all sorts of things. The important thing is to pick the place that is best for you as an individual!"

Before her next meeting with Wes, Shari did a good deal of research into the residential facilities in the area. In the end, she was able to develop a list of some nine different facilities, each described in terms of its population, programs, client problems, supervision, and other significant features. When Wes arrived, she and he began to explore the alternatives reflected on this list. They did this in terms of a specific set of personal values that Shari helped Wes to develop: such values as living in an uncrowded situation, living with people his own age, and so on.

Given Wes's clearly stated values and the information that Shari had gathered, the two were able to make considerable progress. Westwood House and several other facilities were eliminated because their client populations were largely heroin addicts undergoing a methadone maintenance treatment. Since Wes's drugs-of-choice had been marijuana and "speed," such facilities really didn't seem appropriate. Other facilities were eliminated because of one or another of Wes's own personal values. In the end, one facility — a group home called the Downey House — emerged as the clear favorite.

But then the powers-that-be threw a monkey wrench into Wes's and Shari's careful plans: Downey House, they learned, had just lost part of its funding and was thus unable to accept any more new residents!

This was a setback. Fortunately, Shari knew how to deal with it. None of Wes's other alternatives was really favorable. But one — a place called Exodus House — had posed only one significant problem. Wes placed a lot of value on privacy; and Exodus House generally placed new residents in four-bed dormitory rooms.

Would it be possible, Shari wondered, to modify this particular alternative — to get Wes a private room at Exodus House?

It was certainly worth a try. So Shari contacted the director of Exodus House and outlined Wes's situation and the crucial need for privacy.

"Well ....." The director considered the matter. "We usually can't handle requests for private rooms. As it happens, however, we are not very full at this particular time. We've been moving some of our present residents into singles, and I don't see any reason why we couldn't give Wes a single as well."

Full of fresh excitement, Shari and Wes recycled the decision-making process to include this new information. Sure enough — the possibility of privacy at Exodus House transformed this setting into the preferred and clearly favorable alternative for Wes!

"That's it, then," Wes said, real pleasure in his voice. "Man, I'm glad you thought to check out the chances for a single at Exodus! I really would have been crawling up the walls at some place like Westwood!"

"It feels good to know you've chosen the best spot for your own particular situation," Shari responded. "And that positive feeling makes a lot of difference to your chances!"

Shari wasn't kidding. She knew that the confidence Wes felt about his stay at Exodus House was a crucial ingredient in his overall program of treatment. Finding himself in a totally inappropriate facility, he might well have used this as an excuse to get back into drugs. "Man, this just isn't where my head is at!" But, like Shari, Wes himself knew that Exodus House represented his best possible option. And knowing this, he would also know that if he didn't make it here, he probably couldn't make it anywhere.

But Wes would make it. For he had Shari to work with him, and Shari wasn't about to take a single chance with her young client.

Chapter 3 ARRANGING FOR THE CLIENT'S UTILIZATION OF THE COMMUNITY RESOURCE

ARRANGING FOR THE CLIENT'S UTILIZATION OF THE COMMUNITY RESOURCE: AN UNSKILLED APPROACH

Up to now, Pam had worked carefully and effectively with Larry. Given his background and situation, she knew it would be unproductive if he found himself involved in a program that didn't really fit his own needs. For this reason, she had been particularly conscientious in gathering information about specific employment training programs and in helping Larry explore the alternatives and choose the best program for his own purposes.

"This really sounds great." Larry's enthusiastic endorsement of the C.E.T.A. training program they had selected rewarded Pam for her time and effort. Larry obviously felt very good about the whole thing.

The particular program in which Larry would be involved was designed to give him the skills he would need to find full-time work as a hospital orderly. Larry found the possibility of working in this area very exciting. He was a moody, often tense individual whose volatile temper had cost him a number of different jobs in the past. Now he yearned for a type of employment he could really count on, a job that would be both steady and interesting. The C.E.T.A. program promised to move him quickly toward just such a job.

Noting Larry's enthusiastic commitment to the program he had chosen, Pam allowed herself to relax. He would be fine, she felt. Now maybe she could shift her concentration to some of her other clients. Pam's secretary had already contacted the C.E.T.A. people to arrange for Larry's initial visit. Having made sure that Larry knew when and where he should go on Monday to begin the program and having scheduled a follow-up session with him, Pam saw him off.

Alas, she should not have abandoned Larry quite so soon. In particular, she should have explored the C.E.T.A. program itself a bit more and been careful to prepare both Larry and the program's instructor for Larry's involvement. For the instructor, it turned out, was a gruff, ex-military type who made much of exercising his authority. And Larry, as Pam well knew, had a long history of difficulty in dealing with authoritarian figures.

But Pam did not follow through in preparing either Larry or the instructor. She simply sent Larry off, assuming that all would be well. But all was most definitely not well.

Within ten minutes of Larry's entrance into the program the next Monday, he and the instructor had already locked horns over the matter of where Larry would sit. Losing this particular struggle, Larry was in a bad humor for the rest of the class. Still, he might have hung on if the instructor hadn't taken him aside as the first session was ending.

"Son, I've been keeping my eye on you," the older man said in the manner of a general addressing a rebellious soldier. "You're going to have to stay on the ball if you want to keep up in here. And that means you're going to have to have a positive attitude!"

"Oh yeah?" Larry's anger was evident. "What's wrong with my attitude?"

"Well, for one thing, you've done nothing but sneer at me from the back of the room since you came in." The instructor glared down at Larry. "I believe I heard you laugh several times as well."

"Is that right?" Larry was furious. "Well, maybe it's because I thought you were pretty funny, old man!"

Things only got worse after that. The argument ended with Larry stalking out of the room and slamming the door behind him. He simply could not deal with the crusty instructor.

But he could have dealt with him — and the instructor could have worked with Larry more effectively — if Pam had thought to prepare both of them in advance. Sure, Larry was plagued by a lack of self-control. And sure, the instructor was a man preoccupied by his own authority. But in the end, the responsibility for the failure was Pam's. She could have developed programs for each of them. Failing to do so, she paved the way for Larry's inevitable departure.

At this point, the practitioner has selected the resource to meet the client's needs. The next step involves connecting the client to the resource. The skills of arranging to utilize the preferred resource include: (1) preparing to make the resource aware of the client's need; (2) obtaining the agreement of the resource to provide service; (3) finalizing the arrangements to utilize the resource; and (4) developing a program to utilize the resource. The skills and related subskills for arranging to utilize the preferred resource are portrayed in Table 32.

Table 32. The Skills and Subskills of Arranging for the Client's Utilization of the Community Resource

I. PREPARING TO MAKE THE RESOURCE AWARE OF THE CLIENT'S NEED

II. OBTAINING THE AGREEMENT OF THE RESOURCE TO PROVIDE SERVICE

   A. Identifying the advantages to the resource of serving the client
   B. Identifying the client's assets
   C. Anticipating the resource's objections

III. FINALIZING THE ARRANGEMENTS TO UTILIZE THE RESOURCE

   A. Determining client favorability scales for alternatives
   B. Determining resource favorability scales for alternatives
   C. Preparing a written agreement

IV. DEVELOPING A PROGRAM TO UTILIZE THE RESOURCE

   A. Identifying potential problems and goals
   B. Developing program steps
   C. Identifying program responsibility

PREPARING TO MAKE THE RESOURCE AWARE OF THE CLIENT'S NEED

To prepare for the initial contact with the preferred resource, the practitioner answers five essential questions: First, the practitioner formulates the referral goal, *a clear statement of the client outcome being requested from the resource.* It is helpful for practitioners who refer clients to community resources to make certain that they provide a detailed behavioral statement of what is desired from the community resource. Because the purpose of most referrals is to request the community resource to work toward specific skill outcomes, the practitioner defines the need of the client as a need to develop a skill. For example, in making rehabilitation referrals, the practitioner does not simply request such services as "work adjustment training" or "short-term therapy." The referral is based on a prior rehabilitation diagnosis and, thus, is a request for certain skill outcomes — such as "improved ability to converse with coworkers" or "improved ability to differentially reinforce spouse and children." In addition, the referral can focus on the client's skill strengths and deficits in relation to present and potential environmental settings. Diagnostic labels, elaborate descriptions of symptomatology, and hypotheses tied to various psychotherapeutic theories have little relevance to the attainment of rehabilitation goals and thus are unimportant pieces of referral information.

Second, the practitioner identifies the program characteristics that are desired for the client. This descriptive statement of the service vehicle for achieving the referral objective is derived from the values and preferences clarified prior to the decision making. Table 31 provides an example of the service characteristics in the case of John.

Third, the practitioner prepares a clear introductory statement of who he or she is. The statement can include the practitioner's name, role, and agency represented.

Fourth, the practitioner prepares a clear introductory statement of who the client is. In providing a picture of the client, the practitioner can determine what facts are appropriate to share with the new resource. At a minimum, a brief statement of the client's problem will need to be shared.

Fifth, the practitioner clearly expresses why this specific resource is being contacted. The practitioner may compose a statement explaining how the resource was selected to meet the needs of the client. The statement may also include a description of the decision-making values in which the preferred resource alternative scored relatively high.

Practice Situations

Table 33 provides an example of information prepared by John's practitioner prior to contact with the preferred resource. As an initial practice exercise, assume that Katherine and her practitioner have decided to use a modified C.E.T.A. program for their job placement agency. The preferred modified resource for Katherine includes arranging for Katherine to be assigned to a specific C.E.T.A counselor and to receive job placement training from a local continuing education program. First, restate Katherine's referral goal. When you have completed the statement of her referral goal, answer the remaining preparatory questions using a format similar to Table 33.

Table 33. Preparing to Make the Resource Aware of the Client's Need (John)

Question	Answer
What is the client's referral goal?	To be educated at the bachelor level
What service characteristics are required?	(Listed in Table 31)
Who am I?	Martha Jones, Psychiatric Rehabilitation Counselor at the George City Community Mental Health Center
Who is the client?	John is a young man who has experienced past difficulties in completing educational programs when living away from home. John is looking for a good *local* program that will allow him to maintain his family support.
Why was the resource chosen?	Opportunities for interaction with instructors, course compatibility with John's interests, the opportunity to earn a bachelor's degree, and the fact that John fits the eligibility requirements.

OBTAINING THE AGREEMENT OF THE RESOURCE TO PROVIDE SERVICE

After the five awareness questions have been completed, the second major skill in arranging for the client's utilization of the resource is obtaining the agreement of the resource to provide the service. In many instances, this is a simple task. The resource exists and is designed to provide the service requested. It has openings available and is familiar with the kinds of needs for which the client is being referred. In these instances, all that is needed by the practitioner is information similar to the type provided in Table 33. In some instances, however, the referral will require more effort by the practitioner and involve explaining to the resource the benefits of helping the client. For example, when the preferred resource has been chosen as a result of the modification of a resource alternative, the practitioner must work to get the agreement of the resource to provide the modified service to the client.

Another common situation is one in which the practitioner is limited in the psychiatric rehabilitation options available to meet a client's needs. Here it becomes necessary for the practitioner to select a resource that is not designated for psychiatric rehabilitation purposes. For example, when the practitioner needs an educational tutor to help a client learn to read English, a local community action program may be the only alternative. The practitioner will need to persuade the community action program to designate a reading tutor to work with the psychiatric rehabilitation client. It may require special skills to negotiate an agreement with this program to provide services to this "different" type of client.

Obtaining the agreement of the resource involves three subskills: (1) identifying the advantages to the resource of serving the client; (2) identifying the client's assets; and (3) anticipating the resource's objections. By performing these particular steps, the practitioner can become a more skillful "advocate" for the client.

IDENTIFYING THE ADVANTAGES TO THE RESOURCE

In identifying advantages to the resource, the practitioner explains how the resource can benefit by providing the service to the client. Typical benefits or advantages that can be presented to a resource include: (1) generating new funds; (2) receiving positive publicity; (3) increasing goodwill; (4) reducing work load; (5) realizing the resource's mandate or mission; (6) increasing productivity-efficiency; and (7) saving money. The practitioner can begin by listing the advantages that specifically apply to the preferred resource. To list these advantages, the practitioner can first identify from the list of seven typical benefits any that might result from the resource agreeing to help the client. Second, the practitioner can add to the list any other advantages that apply to the particular resource. An approach to generating advantages to the resource is to think about the resource's values and decide how helping the client can contribute to attainment of these values. Here, a knowledge of the resource's mission and purpose is helpful.

After the list of advantages is completed, the practitioner describes how each identified advantage can be attained. For example, if John's practitioner identified "publicity" as an advantage for the university, then a description of how it can be achieved might include the practitioner's submission of an article to the local newspaper. Table 34 presents a list of the advantages that John and his practitioner identified and described.

Practice Situations

As a practice exercise, using a format similar to Table 34, list and describe the advantages to the C.E.T.A. program of agreeing to allow Katherine to be seen by the counselor with the reputation for being most skilled in forming a good counseling relationship with her clients.

Table 34. Advantages to the Resource (John)

Advantage	How Achieved
Publicity	John's practitioner will submit an article to the local newspaper.
Realizing stated university objectives	Meeting special needs of community residents is one of the priorities of the Board of Directors as stated in the Annual Report and university catalogue.
Generating new funds	With present decrease in number of students, programs for psychiatric rehabilitation clients supported by the State Rehabilitation Department may be a new source of students and revenue.
Student internships	Practitioner's agency will be willing to negotiate internship placements for university students in human service area.

IDENTIFYING THE CLIENT'S ASSETS

The second subskill in persuading the resource to accept the client is to present the client's assets. The assets of the client, especially those that relate to achieving the overall program goal, will be important in encouraging the resource to help the client. The practitioner can begin by listing the assets or strengths of the client. Many of these assets can come from the diagnostic planning process (Book 1: *The Skills of Diagnostic Planning*) that operationalized the client's assets in relation to her or his specific living, learning, and working environments. The practitioner may add any client assets that have become apparent during community service coordination.

Once the list of assets is complete, the practitioner will want to write a description of how the client's assets provide "assurances" that the referral goal can be achieved. For example, the fact that John is in good physical condition assures that he has the energy to study and attend classes. The "environmental asset" of his sister's support assures that he will have the physical surroundings conducive to studying at home. Table 35 presents the list of John's assets and shows how they help assure his achieving his overall referral goal.

Table 35. Assets and Related Assurances (John)

Asset	Type	Assurance
Ability to get up in morning	Physical	Assures he can make it to class on time
Physical condition	Physical	Assures he has energy to study and attend classes
Ability to relate to instructors	Emotional	Assures he can get along with instructors
Ability to make friends	Emotional	Assures he can make friends with other students and fit into the university environment
Reading speed	Intellectual	Assures he can complete reading assignments quickly
Listening ability	Intellectual	Assures he can hear what instructors have said during class
Transportation	Environmental	Assures he can get to school for classes
Sister's support	Environmental	Assures he has space, quiet, and cooperation needed to study at home

Practice Situations

Table 36 presents a list of Katherine's assets. Try to show how each of these assets will help ensure that Katherine will achieve her overall referral goal.

Table 36. Assets and Related Assurances (Katherine)

Asset	Type	Assurance
Good grooming	Physical	
Ability to introduce self well to new persons	Emotional	
Good memory	Intellectual	
Husband's encouragement	Environmental	

ANTICIPATING THE RESOURCE'S OBJECTIONS

Although the practitioner may present the advantages to the resource and outline the client's assets, the resource may still be reluctant to provide service. The practitioner, therefore, will want to be prepared to respond to the objections of the resource. Objections may stem from client deficits or liabilities (e.g., lack of social skills) or from the resource's own situation (e.g., staff resistance to working with psychiatric patients). To overcome objections, the practitioner can employ a number of strategies. One strategy is to turn a client liability into an asset. For example, a potential liability for John is that he was a drug user. This can be turned into an asset by pointing out John's successful response to treatment and his deep commitment to not using drugs. A second strategy is to compensate for a liability by showing how other client characteristics help alleviate that particular liability. For example, another potential liability for John is that he was a psychiatric patient. The university might object that his past hospitalizations would upset other students. In response to this objection, the practitioner might point out that John's outgoing and friendly manner has helped him in the past to win many friends. A third strategy is to deny that the liability is critical. This involves showing that the resource's fears will not materialize. For example, in John's case, the university might be concerned that its instructors are not prepared to meet the needs of a psychiatrically disabled student. The practitioner might counter this objection by indicating that John will continue to rely on his practitioner for help with his personal problems and make only appropriate demands on his instructors.

To prepare for the potential objections of the resource, the practitioner needs to anticipate the objections. The practitioner can begin by listing the possible objections the resource may have to helping the client. To list the objections, the practitioner may review the client's deficits as described during the diagnostic planning process. The practitioner can then select those deficits of which the resource will probably become aware and develop a client liability list. Also, the practitioner will want to be sensitive to any client deficits that might conflict with the resource's situation. For example, if the university has received poor publicity regarding its increase in student drug use, John's practitioner would want to include John's past drug usage on the client liability list. To complete the list, the practitioner includes the resource's problems that might make it difficult to comply with the needs of the client.

The following matrix can be used to generate objections stemming from client and resource liabilities:

	Client	Resource
Physical		
Emotional		
Intellectual		

79

Physical liabilities are either behavioral inabilities or liabilities physically affecting the client or the resource. For example, the resource's lack of empty beds would be a physical liability. Emotional liabilities involve the feelings of the client or resource staff or their inability to relate well to each other. For example, the resource staff's fear of working with psychiatric patients would be an emotional liability. Finally, intellectual liabilities primarily involve thinking or mental behavior. For example, the resource staff's lack of knowledge about drug usage would be an intellectual liability.

Once the list of client and resource liabilities is complete, the practitioner will want to write an accompanying statement of the strategy for handling each of the liabilities. Table 37 presents the list of John's liabilities and a strategy statement for each.

Table 37. Liabilities and Strategy Statements (John)

Liability	Strategy	Strategy Statement
Past drug usage	Turn liability into asset	As a result of rehabilitation, John is committed to not using drugs.
Past psychiatric patient	Liability compensation	John's outgoing and friendly manner will help him overcome anxiety of other students and win friends.
Past record of dropping out of school programs	Turn liability into asset	As result of treatment, John is committed to completing an educational program. Also, John is now aware of reasons for past dropouts and has worked hard to develop skills to counteract these past reasons.
Instructors' lack of experience with psychiatrically disabled clients	Deny liability	John will be using practitioner, not instructors, for rehabilitation support. Also, in past, he has made appropriate demands of instructors.
University's lack of experience in getting internships	Deny liability	University has had internship experiences in graduate programs (e.g., psychology). Practitioner can help get John internship placements if university will participate.

Having completed the preparation to make the resource aware of the client and to persuade the resource to accept the client, the practitioner is ready to contact the resource. The practitioner can begin by presenting him or herself, presenting the client's overall referral goal and needed services, and sharing with the resource the reasons it has been chosen (i.e., the basic information summarized in Table 33). If the resource does not agree to accept the client, the practitioner can then proceed to persuade the resource by: (1) presenting the advantages of accepting the client; (2) presenting the client's assets and showing how they assure successful achievement of the referral goal; and (3) eliciting and overcoming the resource's objections. If the resource does not share its objections to helping the client, the practitioner can use the interviewing skills described in Book 1 of this series (*The Skills of Diagnostic Planning*) to attempt to elicit potential objections. Once the resource agrees to provide service, the practitioner can proceed to negotiate the details of the agreement to provide service.

In some instances, the resource will either delay making a decision or refuse service to the client. At this point, the practitioner will want to be prepared with a response that keeps open the possibility of further discussion with the resource. If the resource delays its decision, the practitioner can request any of the following actions to discuss the referral further: (1) another meeting with the resource representative; (2) a meeting with the resource representative's colleagues; or (3) a telephone call or visit within a short period. The purpose of requesting additional opportunities to discuss the referral is to give the practitioner an opportunity to prepare additional persuasive responses (e.g., reasons that will overcome objections, a new list of client assets).

If the resource decides negatively, the practitioner may either work to open up additional opportunities to discuss the referral or attempt to engage the resource in finding another resource to help the client. Possible responses include: (1) a request to call back within a short period in case there has been a change in the decision; (2) a request that the resource telephone another resource that might be able to help the client; or (3) a request that the resource provide the name of another resource that might be able to help the client. The purpose of these responses is twofold: to find an alternative resource to help the client and to try to end with a positive relationship with the resource. When the resource decides negatively and no other resource can provide the service to the client, the practitioner can recycle the decision-making process in order to identify a new preferred resource. If the resource decides to help the client, however, the final step in obtaining the commitment of the resource is to secure the best possible services for the client.

Practice Situations

Table 38 presents a list of Katherine's liabilities. Write a strategy statement for each liability. Set up a role play with a colleague in which you attempt to obtain the commitment of the C.E.T.A. resource to accept Katherine for services. Use a system similar to the one just described. First present yourself and the client's overall referral goal and needed services to the resource. Share with the resource the reasons it was chosen. If necessary, persuade a reluctant resource by presenting the advantages to the resource, showing how the client's assets assure successful achievement of the referral goal, and eliciting and overcoming the resource's objections. If the "role player" resource remains negative, attempt to conclude the interview with a positive note.

Table 38. Liabilities and Strategy Statements (Katherine)

Liability	Strategy	Strategy Statement
Past unemployment record (unemployed for past six years)		
Past psychiatric hospitalizations		
The specific C.E.T.A. counselor requested overloaded with cases		

OBTAINING THE AGREEMENT OF THE RESOURCE TO PROVIDE SERVICE: A SUMMARY

Goal: To obtain the resource's commitment to providing the necessary service to the client

1. Identify the advantages to the resource of serving the client.
2. Identify the client's assets. Select the assets from previously collected diagnostic data as well as information collected during the community support coordination process.
3. Anticipate the resource's objections: (a) identify potential client and resource liabilities; (b) write a strategy statement for each liability.

FINALIZING THE ARRANGEMENTS TO UTILIZE THE RESOURCE

In finalizing the arrangements for using the resource, the practitioner negotiates an agreement that specifies the referral goal and the services the client is to receive relevant to the goal. The negotiation develops a clear picture or statement of the service to be provided to the client and the context in which it is to be provided. An agreement ensures that the client will receive appropriate help from the resource and serves as a guide for later monitoring of the resource. Although a written agreement is not legally binding, it specifies the service to be provided to the client. As was mentioned previously, many times the negotiation of an agreement is fairly straightforward. The referral agreement, if written, can be based on the initial referral information (similar to the example in Table 33).

However, there are also instances in which the agreement negotiations are more complex. This is usually the case when the practitioner is trying to obtain some "special" arrangement with the resource, such as a modification of the alternative's standard operating procedures. For example, John's practitioner was pleased that, after persuasive efforts, the university expressed openness to accepting John and modifying the course requirements and internship possibilities. Yet neither the specific changes in course requirements and internships nor the terms of the acceptance had been clarified. Acceptance terms might range from unconditional acceptance to the requirement that John successfully complete prerequisite courses. Before meeting with the university personnel to negotiate the agreement, therefore, John's practitioner defined three issues to be negotiated: (1) acceptance terms; (2) course requirements; and (3) internship opportunities. The establishment in an agreement format of these issues would serve to "firm up" the kind of service John required from the university.

Finalizing arrangements for using a resource proceeds through three substeps: (1) determining client favorability scales for alternatives; (2) determining resource favorability scales for alternatives; and (3) preparing a written agreement.

DETERMINING CLIENT FAVORABILITY SCALES FOR ALTERNATIVES

Determining client favorability scales for alternatives means understanding different alternatives from the client's perspective.

When exploring agreement alternatives, the practitioner determines how favorable each alternative is to the client. Using a variation on the decision-making skills described in Chapter 2, the practitioner can develop a favorability scale for each agreement issue — ranging from very favorable (level 5) to minimally acceptable (level 1). It simply makes good negotiating sense for the practitioner, if possible, to have anticipated this range of possible agreement options *before* the actual negotiation takes place. This is not to say that unanticipated possibilities will not occur. This preparation merely improves the practitioner's competence in advocating for the best possibilities for the client.

The first step is to explore the alternative agreements and choose the most favorable alternative for the client. The most favorable alternative would be designated level 5 and placed at the top of the scale. The second step is to explore the remaining alternatives and choose the alternative that would be minimally acceptable in helping the client achieve the goal. This alternative would be designated level 1 and placed at the bottom of the scale. The third step is to explore the remaining alternatives and choose the one that could be considered moderately favorable. The moderately favorable alternative would be designated level 3 and placed in the middle of the scale. The fourth step is to consider whether an alternative falls between very favorable and moderately favorable for the client. If so, this alternative is designated favorable and placed at level 4 on the scale. Finally, the practitioner considers whether an alternative falls between moderately favorable and minimally acceptable to the client. If so, the alternative would be characterized as acceptable and placed at level 2 on the scale. Obviously, there will be instances when there are not five levels of favorability for each issue to be negotiated. The key concern is for the practitioner to take the time to consider as many possibilities as he or she can before the actual negotiations take place.

The resulting client favorability scale can have from two to five levels that define how favorable the possible alternative agreements are to the client. Table 39 presents the favorability scales for the three agreement issues John's practitioner specified as negotiable.

Practice Situations

Table 40 presents some sample agreement issues for Katherine. Complete the favorability scales presented in Table 40 for the agreement issues that might be relevant in negotiations for Katherine's use of the C.E.T.A. program.

Table 39. Client Favorability Scales for Agreement Issues (John)

Agreement Issue	Level	Favorability Scale
Acceptance terms	5	Unconditional
	4	Conditional acceptance until successful completion of first year
	3	College Boards or ACT results
	2	Successful completion of specific course
	1	Successful completion of prerequisite courses
Course requirements	5	None
	4	Negotiable with John
	3	At least three alternatives for each requirement
	2	Composition only
	1	Language and composition only
Internship opportunities	5	50 percent or more of course work
	4	36–49 percent of course work
	3	20–35 percent of course work
	2	10–19 percent of course work
	1	Less than 10 percent of course work

Table 40. Client Favorability Scales for Agreement Issues (Katherine)

Agreement Issue	Level	Favorability Scale
Counselor assignment	5	
	4	
	3	
	2	
	1	
Job training	5	
	4	
	3	
	2	
	1	

DETERMINING RESOURCE FAVORABILITY SCALES FOR ALTERNATIVES

Having developed the client's favorability scales for the agreement issues, the practitoner is ready to negotiate an agreement with the resource. The practitioner will seek to have the resource agree to the most favorable terms for the client. However, the practitioner may not always succeed in securing the most favorable agreement. It is important, therefore, for the practitioner to know when to compromise or agree to less favorable terms. The practitioner may wish to develop, either with or without the resource's direct contribution, a favorability scale from the resource's perspective. For example, John's practitioner knew it would be difficult for the university to agree to unconditional acceptance of John; some type of trial period was most favorable to them. By understanding the favorability of the alternatives to both John and the university, the practitioner was prepared to suggest conditional acceptance of John until successful completion of his first year. Table 41 presents the resource favorability scales that John's practitioner developed prior to entering into agreement negotiations with the university. The practitioner developed the favorability scales from the university's perspective before actually hearing the university's view on the agreement issues. The practitioner simply wanted to anticipate the perspective of the resource as closely as possible. A guideline to use in developing a resource's favorability scale is that the more consistent the alternative is with the resource's usual way of functioning, the more favorable it will be to the resource. The purpose of this preparation effort is to make the negotiation process as smooth and as pleasant as possible. The fewer surprises for either party the better. The practitioner's prior knowledge of potential areas of compromise and flexibility will increase her or his ability to negotiate the best possible situation for the client.

Practice Situations

Using Table 42, develop favorability scales for the agreement issues from the C.E.T.A. perspective.

Table 41. Resource Favorability Scales for Agreement Issues (John)

Agreement Issue	Level	Favorability Scale
Acceptance terms	5	Successful completion of prerequisite courses
	4	Conditional acceptance based on first-year grades
	3	Positive College Board or ACT results
	2	Successful completion of specific course
	1	Unconditional
Course requirements	5	Language and composition only
	4	Composition only
	3	At least three alternatives for each requirement
	2	Negotiable with John
	1	None
Internship opportunities	5	None
	4	1–14 percent of course work
	3	15–25 percent of course work
	2	26–35 percent of course work
	1	36 percent or more of course work

Table 42. Resource Favorability Scales for Agreement Issues (Katherine)

Agreement Issue	Level	Favorability Scale
Counselor assignment	5	
	4	
	3	
	2	
	1	
Job training	5	
	4	
	3	
	2	
	1	

PREPARING A WRITTEN AGREEMENT

During the actual meeting to negotiate an agreement, the practitioner will want to use the interviewing skills described in Book 1 of this series *(The Skills of Diagnostic Planning)* in order to elicit the perspective of the resource. Successful negotiations result in the best possible agreement among the practitioner, the client, and the resource.

Stated another way, the agreement is the point of best possible match between the client's and the resource's favorability scales. The practitioner will also need to use the persuasive material developed in the previous section. Presenting the client's assets, showing the advantages to the resource of serving the client, and being able to overcome resource objections are as important in getting the resource to agree to the specifics of the agreement as they are in obtaining the agreement of the resource to help the client. Once the agreement issues have been resolved to the satisfaction of both the resource and the practitioner, a written agreement can be developed and signed. A written agreement ensures that the resource, the client, and the practitioner all understand the agreement. It also helps to ensure the commitment of the resource and the client to completing their parts of the agreement. A written agreement can specify: (1) the responsibilities of those involved (the resource, the client, the practitioner); (2) an operationalized statement of the referral goal and service to be provided, including how the service is to be monitored; (3) the reasons why the service is to be provided; (4) the location where the service is to be provided; and (5) when the service is to be completed.

Table 43 contains the agreement between John and the university. For all the issues, John's practitioner was able to negotiate specific agreements that ranged from somewhat favorable to favorable for John.

After the agreement has been negotiated and written, the first phase of arranging to utilize the preferred resource is completed. The practitioner has obtained the commitment of the resource to provide specific services to the client. The next skill is to develop a program to ensure the effective use of the resource by the client.

Table 43. Sample Written Agreement (John)

June 30, 1977

Ms. Robinson
Massachusetts Department of
  Vocational Rehabilitation
100 Worth Street
Boston, Massachusetts

Dear Ms. Robinson:

In accordance with the university's policy of meeting the educational needs of all residents of Amherst and its commitment to developing the alternative programs necessary to respond to the special needs of students, Amherst State University (A.S.U.) agrees to accept John Williams as a conditional student for the school year 1977-78. The university agrees to accept John into the degree program in Sociology once John successfully completes his first year course work as measured by his maintaining at least a B- or 2.75 grade-point-average. The university also agrees to accept those transfer credits from John's previous college work that are applicable to A.S.U.'s current course work.

A.S.U. also agrees to negotiate course requirements with John as measured by his choice of at least three alternative courses to fulfill each requirement, the only exception being that John will be required to successfully complete the English Composition requirement as measured by obtaining a C or 2.00 grade in the required course.

Additionally, A.S.U. agrees to offer internship experiences as measured by internships representing at least 20 percent of John's course work beginning in the second year, if possible. The Alternative Programs Coordinator will work with [name of counselor] to arrange appropriate internships that are acceptable to the chairman of the Sociology Department and John.

John Williams
John Williams

Robert C. Brown
Admissions Director

Practice Situations

Write an agreement for services to be provided by the C.E.T.A. program for Katherine, filling in the five specific points as presented previously.

FINALIZING THE ARRANGEMENTS TO UTILIZE THE RESOURCE: A SUMMARY

Goal: To negotiate with the resource to obtain the best possible service for the client

1. List the issues to be agreed upon.
2. Determine client favorability scales for agreement issues.
3. Determine resource favorability scales for agreement issues.
4. Negotiate with the resource to resolve the agreement issues.
5. Prepare a written statement.

DEVELOPING A PROGRAM TO UTILIZE THE RESOURCE

Having obtained the resource's agreement to provide the necessary service, the next major skill is to develop a program that will ensure that the client will participate in and benefit from the resource. A program is simply a step-by-step way to achieve a desired goal. It helps to ensure that the course of action will be successfully implemented and enables the client to see exactly what he or she has to do. This in turn allows the client to anticipate points in the implementation process where problems may occur. These points can then be addressed in advance by the client and the practitioner. The second book in this series — *The Skills of Rehabilitation Programming* — describes program development skills in detail. Program development will be only briefly reviewed in this book.

Developing a program to utilize the resource proceeds through the following subskills: (1) identifying potential problems and goals in utilization of the resource; (2) developing program steps: and (3) identifying program responsibility.

The case of Paul will be used to illustrate the process of developing a program to utilize the resource. (Paul's case was used previously to illustrate the skill of operationalizing values; see Table 13.) Paul is in his early twenties, is single, and has had two psychiatric hospitalizations. He is currently unemployed and has a history of a drinking problem. As noted earlier, he had been living with his parents at the time of his last admission, but Paul and his practitioner had decided that he should explore an alternative living situation. In the diagnostic plan they jointly developed, it was decided that Paul needed a living environment where there would be supervision available to assist him in mastering the activities of daily living and managing his own behavior. His goal, then, was to identify the best place where he could live. Because Paul and his practitioner felt that one year of supervised living would be sufficient for Paul to master skills required to live on his own, the placement sought was for one year's time. Using the skills of selecting the preferred community resource, Paul and his practitioner identified the Green House as the best place for him. Now that the preferred resource had been chosen, it was possible to identify the overall referral goal more specifically. Thus, Paul's overall referral goal became: "to live at Green House for one year."

IDENTIFYING POTENTIAL PROBLEMS AND GOALS

In identifying problems and goals in using the resource, the practitioner will want to plan for problems that may hinder the client's successful utilization of the resource. The practitioner can begin by identifying those difficulties that could prevent the client from reaching the referral goal. During diagnostic planning and rehabilitation programming the practitioner and client will have successfully identified and treated a number of client deficits. Any remaining deficit behaviors that will hinder the client's utilization of the resource need to be improved. Here the practitioner can pose the question: *What deficits exist in the client and/or the resource that might lead to failure in the use of the resource?* The following matrix can be used for expanding possible problems:

	Client Problems	*Resource Problems*
Physical		
Emotional-interpersonal		
Intellectual		

This book considers personnel as part of the resource. Therefore, just as with the client, the resource may include physical, emotional-interpersonal, and intellectual problems.

For example, the practitioner and Paul identified two problems that might interfere with Paul's successful use of Green House. The first was Paul's difficulty in constructively disagreeing with others; the second was that the treatment personnel at Green House did not know Paul well. Note that the practitioner skilled in community service coordination needs to consider not only client problems *but also potential resource problems*. This step of identifying potential resource problems is particularly important when using resources that have had little experience in working with psychiatrically disabled clients. Yet even professionals and agencies with established track records in dealing with psychiatrically disabled clients may still need specific programs or program steps developed for certain clients. Community resources are often geared for the psychiatrically disabled client *in general*. The referring practitioner may be able to contribute to the community resource's preparation for a *particular* client.

Once the client and resource problems have been identified, the next step is to operationalize the resource-use problem. The components that are required for operationalizing the problem are as follows:

1. Who has the problem?	Tell who has the problem.
2. What is the problem?	State the problem.
3. What are observable signs?	Tell the observable symptoms that describe the problem.
4. How is it to be measured?	Use time (amount of time), frequency (number of times), and/or amount to quantify the problem.
5. When and where does the problem occur?	Tell the conditions under which the problem occurs.

For example, the problems that are relevant to Paul's use of Green House might be operationalized as follows:

Problem 1: Paul cannot discuss differences constructively as measured by the percentage of time he ends up shouting or pouting when he has a disagreement with someone at home or work.

Problem 2: Green House treatment personnel do not know Paul, as measured by the number of Paul's observable behaviors that they can use to monitor the adequacy of Paul's progress.

Based on this operationalization of the problem, the current functioning of the client and/or the resource can be assessed and observable resource-use goals set. An example of how this may be accomplished is presented in Table 44. As suggested by the table, the first step in the operationalization process is to explore and assess the client's or resource's present functioning on the deficit behavior. The resource-use goal is then specified by exploring and assessing the functioning that needs to be achieved by the client or resource.

Table 44. Client Assessment Chart for Operationalized Resource-Use Problems (Paul)

Operationalized Problem	Present Functioning	Resource-Use Goal
Percentage of time Paul ends up shouting or pouting about a disagreement	30–40	10 or less
Use of observable behaviors to monitor adequacy of Paul's progress	None	Use of all known behaviors

Practice Situations

As a practice exercise, work with Mary, whose initial problem was that she could not occupy her days and evenings with anything but watching television. Her goal was to spend at least five hours a week in group leisure-time activities outside her home. Imagine that Mary had decided to start filling her leisure time by enrolling in the adult education crafts program offered by the local high school. Mary has two problems that could interfere with her effective use of this resource. First, she does not know how to use the public transportation system that will allow her to get from her home to the school. Second, even though she would like to, she does not know how to socialize with other people. In fact, she does not know how to greet people. Begin the exercise by using this information to specify an overall referral goal for Mary. Then, operationalize her two resource-use problems, assess her present functioning, and specify her resource-use goals. Use a format similar to Table 44. Also, practice operationalizing resource-use problems, assessing present functioning, and developing resource-use goals with a client or a friend.

DEVELOPING PROGRAM STEPS

Having set the resource-use goals, the next task is to develop the steps that will lead to attainment of the goal. To do this, the practitioner and/or the client first brainstorm the steps involved. After the steps have been brainstormed, they need to be sequenced. In other words, they need to be ordered from the first step to the last step.

Finally, where it is appropriate, the practitioner develops and sequences the necessary secondary steps. To be functional, a program includes only steps that the client can complete. Therefore, the number and the size of the steps will vary according to the client's functioning in the particular area. For example, to give directions or steps for

93

reaching an address to a person familiar with the geographic area, one might simply say, "I'm at two-thirty-four Marlboro Street. Just turn left at the intersection of Main and Marlboro, and it's the fourth house on the left." But if the person was not at all familiar with the area, more detailed directions or steps would be necessary (e.g., how to get to Main Street, how to recognize the intersection of Main Street and Marlboro Street). In other words, when all the steps are developed, the person who is to use the program should be able to look at each step and complete it successfully. Examples of the steps in the programs used to help Paul are presented in Tables 45 and 46. The steps in the disagreement program are for Paul to follow under the guidance of the practitioner. The steps to prepare treatment personnel at the Green House are for the practitioner to follow.

Table 45. Resource-Use Program (Paul)

Resource-use goal: Shout or pout less than ten percent of the time when there is a disagreement.

Brainstorm steps:

Present own side in civil tone.
Listen to other's side.
Suggest compromise, if possible.

Pay attention to other.
Make sure other understands my side.
Practice in discussions with practitioner.
Practice in discussions in daily life.

Sequence steps:

1. Pay attention.
2. Listen to other's side.
3. Present my side civilly.

4. Make sure other understands my side.
5. Suggest compromise, if possible.
6. Practice in discussions with practitioner.
7. Practice in discussions in daily life.

Develop and sequence secondary steps:

1. Pay attention
   a. Face other person squarely.
   b. Look at other person's face.

2. Listen to other's side.
   a. Summarize what other said in my head.
   b. Reflect what other said, using phrase such as "You're saying _____ ."
   c. Clarify any errors on my part.
   d. Ask relevant questions about other's point of view.

3. Present my side civilly.
   a. State what I think or feel.
   b. State why I think or feel that.

4. Make sure other understands my side.
   a. Ask if other has any questions about what I said.
   b. Ask if other would mind summarizing what he/she understood me to say, e.g., "I don't always say things just the way I want. Would you mind just summarizing what you think I've said to you about this?"

5. Suggest compromise, if possible.
   a. Ask if other has any ideas about how we might compromise.
   b. Suggest any ideas on compromise of my own.

6. Practice in discussions with practitioner.
   a. Practice paying attention.
   b. Practice listening to other's side.
   c. Practice presenting my side civilly.
   d. Practice making sure other understands my side.
   e. Practice suggesting compromise.

7. Practice in discussions in daily life.
   a. Practice paying attention.
   b. Practice listening to other's side.
   c. Practice presenting my side civilly.
   d. Practice making sure other understands my side.
   e. Practice suggesting compromise.

Table 46. Resource-Use Program (Practitioner)

Resource-use goal: Get treatment personnel at Green House to monitor Paul, using all behaviors that are known to me.

Brainstorm steps:

Draw up list of critical behaviors known to me.
Develop rating form.
Make arrangements for feedback.

Get input from treatment staff about using instrument.
Revise instrument so that it is useful to staff.

Sequence steps:

1. Draw up list of critical behaviors known to me.
2. Develop rating form.
3. Get input from treatment staff about using instrument.

4. Revise instrument.
5. Make arrangements for feedback.

Develop and sequence secondary steps:

1. Draw up list of critical behaviors known to me.
2. Develop rating form.
3. Get input from treatment staff about using instrument.
    a. Ask what behaviors they can monitor.
    b. Ask procedures they would use.

4. Revise instrument.
5. Make arrangements for feedback.
    a. Determine frequency of feedback.
    b. Determine method by which report will be made.

Practice Situations

For each of the resource-use goals you specified for Mary, develop steps to reach them. Use a format similar to Tables 45 and 46. When you have completed the practice excercise with Mary, develop steps to a resource-use goal with a client or friend.

IDENTIFYING PROGRAM RESPONSIBILITY

Identifying program responsibility specifies who is to complete the program steps as defined. There are essentially three types of programs for the utilization of a community resource. The first type is a *client program where the practitioner is responsible* for the delivery of the program steps to the client, who in turn will follow the steps. This type of program is often appropriate when the practitioner wishes to prepare the client for the new resource. Paul's program for less shouting or pouting is an example of this type of program. Paul's practitioner accepts responsibility for developing the program and helping Paul to implement it.

The second type is a *client program where the staff at the resource is responsible* for the client's implementation of the program steps. If Paul's practitioner either developed Paul's program for reduced shouting with the staff at Green House or gave the program to the Green House staff to evaluate and modify, the same program could become an example of the second type.

Finally, there are *practitioner programs where the practitioner develops a program for either the resource staff or him or herself to follow* (either with the resource staff or independently). The practitioner or the resource staff assumes responsibility for the program and follows the steps defined in the program. In this type of program, the practitioner can act in a consulting capacity to facilitate the resource's ability to help the client. The program for Paul's practitioner to help Green House monitor Paul is an example of the third type of program.

DEVELOPING A PROGRAM TO UTILIZE THE RESOURCE: A SUMMARY

Goal: To ensure that the client participates in and benefits from utilization of the resource

1. Identify potential problems and goals in utilization of the resource.

2. Develop program steps.

3. Identify program responsibility.

ARRANGING FOR THE CLIENT'S UTILIZATION OF THE COMMUNITY RESOURCE: A SKILLED APPROACH

Felipe knew that the choice confronting Elda was a crucial one. Things had not been going well for her. She had managed to get into far more than her share of trouble. Now everything hung in the balance. She could either remain in the hospital on weekends, a move guaranteed to disrupt not only her own life but the lives of her family even more than they had already been disrupted. Or she could start spending weekends at home, a possibility full of risk for both Elda and her husband and small children with whom she lived.

Felipe moved cautiously. He helped Elda to lay out her alternatives in clear-cut terms. It was critically important that she understand the assets and liabilities of both ways of spending weekends. They spent a long time together exploring and evaluating the two possibilities. In the end, both Felipe and his client felt that the best decision involved Elda going home on weekends and returning to the hospital during the week.

But Felipe knew that his real work was just beginning. If Elda was going to make it, she was going to have to know just what her goals were and just how she could reach them.

"Like I told you before, one of my biggest problems is just finding the time to do all the things I need to do at home," Elda told Felipe. And so he helped her set a specific goal for herself which involved organizing necessary weekend tasks in terms of essential rest, available time, and the priority of each task. And he went on to help her develop a careful, step-by-step program with built-in reinforcements that would enable Elda to reach this goal. He then went on to help her set goals and develop appropriate programs in other areas of potential difficulty.

Nor did Felipe stop there. He knew how important significant others could be to any client's progress. One of the people he contacted was Elda's husband, Jess. As the person whose efforts would do most to sustain and promote Elda's achievement of her rehabilitation goals, Jess represented a very real "resource" in his own right.

At first Jess was hesitant. Although he emphasized how much he wanted Elda to work things out, he just wasn't sure he could handle things well at this point if she started coming home on weekends. Felipe understood this hesitancy. But he took pains to make Jess aware of how important the weekends at home were to Elda. He was persuasive in pointing out that progress for Elda would quickly translate into real benefits for Jess himself — he'd have his wife back again! Finally winning Jess over, Felipe worked out an agreement as to how Jess would handle things at home. In effect, this meant helping Jess to set his own goals and develop his own program. All of these goals were simple yet meaningful: such things as "no raising of voices," "at least three specific compliments given to wife each day," and "at least thirty minutes of quiet conversation each night after the children are in bed."

A straightforward objective: to get Elda's husband to serve as a valuable "supporting" resource. Yet even here Felipe had to use specific skills to promote the other man's awareness, to persuade him to help, to get him to agree to specific terms.

In the end, Felipe felt he had done all he could to prepare both Elda and her husband for the former's weekends at home. Still, he knew quite well that the proof of his effectiveness could only be given through Elda's success. Her growth and Felipe's own capability were inextricably twined together.

"It's good — it feels really fine!" Elda's high spirits at their next session were testimony to the success of Felipe's careful planning and preparation. Even at this point he knew that there were no guarantees. He would have to do a great deal of follow-up work with Elda — and with her husband, too — before he could relax and let things take their course. But for now, Felipe felt confident. He had helped Elda avoid a *longer unbroken period of hospitalization, which would have been extremely disruptive for the whole family. He had made it possible for Elda to live at home on weekends, a far more "normal" situation than remaining in the hospital. Most of all, he had helped both Elda and her husband develop the specific goals and programs they needed to make a go of things together during a most difficult time.*

Felipe was no miracle worker. But he knew that in most, if not all situations, careful planning and preparation can do as much good as any miracle.

Chapter 4 SUPPORTING THE CLIENT'S UTILIZATION OF THE COMMUNITY RESOURCE

SUPPORTING THE CLIENT'S UTILIZATION OF THE COMMUNITY RESOURCE: AN UNSKILLED APPROACH

The phone call had jarred Dave and cast a pall over the morning. He had called the McCallurn House, a halfway house for alcoholics, to check on Keith, a client he had referred there the previous week. The director at McCallurn had told Dave that Keith had begun drinking again and had left the house.

A sense of frustration welled up within Dave. Keith had come to the rehabilitation agency from an alcoholic detoxification center. He was in his late twenties and his alcohol problem, although worsening, was not yet chronic.

Keith had agreed that his primary problem was alcohol abuse and that he could benefit from a halfway house where he could sustain a period of sobriety. They had selected McCallurn House because its residents were in Keith's age group. Dave had contacted McCallurn to arrange for a one-month residency for Keith. It was also agreed that Keith would attend AA meetings nightly and could take Antabuse if he felt it necessary.

In thinking back, Dave could recall that, although Keith seemed to recognize his deficits, his motivation did not seem strong enough; his rehabilitation efforts would need to be reinforced and closely supervised. Yet he had done nothing to heighten Keith's motivation or to provide for close supervision at McCallurn House. He had selected a community resource, developed a program, and referred his client without ensuring that the program would be implemented and carried out.

Dave was professional and objective enough to realize that his client's failure was an expression of his failure as a rehabilitation practitioner. Had he followed through and sustained his involvement with and support of Keith at McCallurn, the outcome for Keith might have been different.

After the practitioner has arranged to utilize the preferred community resource, the next stage is to support the client's actual utilization of the resource. Supporting the client's use of the resource ensures that the program steps are implemented by those responsible and that new learning is used to modify any unsuccessful procedures. In effectively supporting the client's use of the resource, the practitioner ensures the successful culmination of community service coordination.

Supporting the client's utilization of the resource includes the following skills: (1) developing time lines for action; (2) developing reinforcers to ensure action; (3) monitoring performance; and (4) modifying the program to improve its effectiveness. The skills of supporting the client's utilization of the resource are presented in Table 47.

Table 47. The Skills of Supporting the Client's Utilization of the Community Resource

---

I.   Developing Time Lines for Action

II.   Developing Reinforcers to Ensure Action

III. Monitoring Performance

IV.   Modifying the Program to Improve Its Effectiveness

DEVELOPING TIME LINES FOR ACTION

Time lines indicate when an action will be initiated and when it will be completed. Time lines allow the practitioner and the client to monitor the progress of resource use. Time lines allow problems to be easily identified, because the passing of an assigned date for action initiation or completion concretely indicates a problem in the use of the resource.

A key guideline for use in establishing time lines is reasonableness. Guidelines that fail to take into consideration the other responsibilities of the implementer of a program step or to properly assess the amount of time needed to complete a resource-use action become impediments in their own right. Thus, two significant questions need to be considered in developing time lines: (1) When can the person responsible for the action reasonably initiate the action? (2) Given the nature of the action, in what amount of time can it reasonably be expected to be completed? Specifically in relation to the latter question, program steps that involve the implementation of a discrete action (e.g., making a telephone call) can be expected to begin and end in the same day. However, a step that involves learning a new skill may require the allocation of a span of time for completion.

Practice Situations

The development of time lines is illustrated in Table 48. As a practice exercise, take the major steps for each of the programs you have developed for Mary and assign time lines. Use a format similar to that depicted in Table 48.

Table 48.   Time Lines for Program Steps (Paul)

Major Steps in Disagreement Program	Starting Date	Completion Date
Pay attention	2/4	2/18
Listen to other's side	2/4	2/18
Present my side civilly	2/4	2/18
Make sure other understands my side	2/11	2/25
Suggest compromise, if possible	2/11	2/25
Practice in discussions with practitioner	2/26	3/3
Practice in discussions in daily life	3/4	3/11
Major Steps in Treatment Staff Program		
List critical behaviors	2/4	2/4
Develop rating form	2/5	2/9
Get input from treatment staff about instrument	2/12	2/12
Revise instrument	2/13	2/13
Make arrangements for feedback	2/18	

DEVELOPING REINFORCERS TO ENSURE ACTION

The practitioner can augment the resource utilization program by identifying reinforcers and linking the reinforcers to program steps. Reinforcers are stimuli that have the effect of motivating action. Sometimes the successful completion of program steps is enough of a reinforcer. However, in some instances, other responsibilities might distract a person to the point where a reinforcer is needed to focus that person's attention on a specific action. In other instances, the goals of the program may become too distant, and the steps leading to the goal may lose their reality. In these cases, reinforcers may be attached to the program steps to heighten their significance.

Developing reinforcers to ensure action involves identifying experiences that are immediate to the action and that will motivate the person implementing the action. An important guideline to use in establishing the reinforcers is that the reinforcer always be based on the perspective of the actor — that is, the reinforcer must be experienced positively or negatively by the person performing the program steps. Another guideline is that anybody, including practitioners, may need a reinforcer. Thus, the practitioner will want to avoid the stereotype that clients require reinforcers because of their inherent weaknesses in acting. Additionally, reinforcers are experiences that can occur immediately after an action. The more proximate the reinforcer is to the event, the more potent it becomes. Still further, reinforcers can be selected so that they are appropriate to the action and likely to occur. In other words, reinforcers need to be realistic. If a reward attached to successful implementation of an action is not realizable (e.g., a trip to Bermuda), or if a punishment attached to the failure to implement an action is excessively harsh or detrimental to the well-being of the individual (e.g., a day without food), the reinforcement process will not be implemented.

An example of the application of reinforcers is provided in the case of Paul. Paul and his practitioner knew that he would need reinforcers attached to the expected actions of practicing his disagreement skills in his daily interactions. One of the things Paul really liked to do was watch TV in the evenings. The practitioner and Paul decided that he could watch TV in the evening only if he daily practiced or applied the behaviors he had learned from his disagreement program.

Practice Situations

Practice assigning reinforcers to Mary's resource utilization program. Of course, you do not have to use the same reinforcer for each step. For example, you might use watching or not watching TV as a reinforcer to completing one step, and going or not going to a restaurant for completing another step. Negative consequences are often the opposite of positive consequences. For example, the client might deprive himself or herself of the privilege of wearing a favorite outfit for some period of time for failure to complete a step. Use these guidelines to develop positive and negative reinforcements for each of the major steps in Mary's program.

MONITORING PERFORMANCE

Time lines and reinforcers provide the structure and dynamic for supporting the client's use of a resource. Monitoring provides a way of ensuring progress in the use of the resource. Monitoring is simply the action of watching to see if what is supposed to happen truly happens.

Monitoring performance proceeds through six substeps: (1)

identifying what is to be monitored; (2) identifying who is to do the monitoring; (3) identifying where the monitoring is to be done; (4) identifying when the monitoring is to be done; (5) identifying how the monitoring is to be done; and (6) identifying how learning from the monitoring is to be shared.

The first step of monitoring performance, identifying what is to be monitored, is already achieved when the practitioner and client design the resource utilization program. Monitoring focuses on specific behaviors defined in the *major steps* of that resource utilization program. The question of who is to do the monitoring is limited to three choices: the client, the practitioner, or the resource personnel. The identification of who is to do the monitoring will depend upon the capacity of the potential monitor to produce reliable and valid observations, the proximity of the monitor to the event, and the willingness of the monitor to cooperate. The context for the monitoring will be where the specific step is to be implemented. When monitoring is to be done requires the identification of specific time and dates. Generally, monitoring is most proximate in time to the event that is to be monitored to ensure accurate and timely reports. Similarly, in determining how monitoring is to be done, the practitioner will want to consider accuracy and timeliness. The procedure most likely reflects what took place but is of a level of complexity that facilitates implementation. Finally, the process of sharing monitoring information ensures accurate communication of feedback in a timely fashion.

Decisions about each of the six steps of monitoring culminate in the development of a written monitoring plan. An example of such a plan is provided in Table 49, again using the case of Paul. Paul's practitioner could see that Paul's progress in carrying out the steps of his disagreement program would require more monitoring than was needed to monitor his own program with the treatment staff. To monitor his own program, the practitioner simply developed a list for checking off the starting and completion of the steps as defined in the time lines. To monitor Paul's progress, however, the practitioner developed an answer to each of the critical questions of monitoring. Table 49 presents the plan that Paul's practitioner developed for monitoring Paul's progress in completing the steps of his disagreement program. The specific behaviors to be monitored come from the major steps of the program. Also, the specification of where and when the monitoring is to occur flows from what is to be monitored. The decision about who is to do the monitoring is based on the previously identified issues. More than one person may be used, depending upon what is being monitored. Independent of who is doing the monitoring, the monitoring results are reported to the person responsible for the implementation of the program step. The most difficult decision concerns how the monitoring can best be done. As can be seen in the example provided in Table 49, a variety of techniques are included: rating forms, audio recordings, video recordings, and direct observations. Again, the device to be used supports accuracy but also is reasonable, given the time, expertise, and equipment resources available for the purposes of monitoring. Although there are a number of ways of sharing learning about progress (e.g., written reports, verbal reports, checklists), the best method is for the person completing the monitoring and the person responsible for implementing the action to meet as often as possible. The more frequent the sharing of new learning, the more opportunity there is to act on the learning.

The monitoring plan used as an example in Table 49 appears quite detailed. However, it is in fact deceptively simple. For many of the steps, the monitoring program is similar. In actual rehabilitation practice, the practitioner would probably only have a few notes as a reminder of any reactions in the monitoring program. Table 49 is an example of all the components of which the practitioner is aware as he or she learns monitoring skills. Once the practitioner learns and practices monitoring skills, it will not be necessary to write such a detailed monitoring plan. However, practitioners will still want to be able to conceptualize such a plan.

Practice Situations

As a practice exercise, design and write a monitoring plan for Mary. Use a format similar to that depicted in Table 49.

MODIFYING THE PROGRAM TO IMPROVE ITS EFFECTIVENESS

The decision as to whether or not to modify the resource utilization program is based on the monitoring results. If the client cannot successfully complete the steps, some kind of modification is required. Aside from very minor modifications such as changing the time line or reinforcement schedules, the practitioner and the client have two major options available. They may either revise a step or build more steps into the process of realizing the goal.

Revising a step of the program requires redefining the difficult step as a subgoal. The program development process is then recycled to brainstorm, sequence, and develop steps to reach the new subgoal. The program is implemented again. The new subgoal and resulting new program represent an intermediate focus in the effort to achieve what, on reassessment, appears to be a longer-term goal.

The other alternative available to the practitioner and client is to build more steps in to the original program. The additional steps would provide a bridge for the client from the last step the client could complete to the step the client is unable to complete.

An example of the modification process is provided in Table 50. In monitoring Paul's disagreement program, the practitioner discovered

Table 49. Monitoring Plan (Paul)

What Step Is to Be Monitored	Who Does the Monitoring	Where the Monitoring Is Done	When the Monitoring Is Done	How the Monitoring Is Done	How Learning from the Monitoring Is Shared
1. Pay attention	Practitioner	Practitioner's office	During skill learning	Observations of practitioner	Verbal feedback from practitioner to client
2. Listen to other's side	Practitioner	Practitioner's office	During and immediately after skill-learning session	Audiotaped role play with practitioner	Listening to tape
3. Present my side civilly	Practitioner	Practitioner's office	During and immediately after skill-learning session	Audiotaped role play with practitioner; rating form	Listening to tape; reviewing practitioner's ratings
4. Make sure other understands my side	Practitioner	Practitioner's office	During and immediately after skill-learning session	Audiotaped role play with practitioner; rating forms; self ratings	Listening to tape; reviewing client's and practitioner's ratings
5. Suggest compromise, if possible	Practitioner	Practitioner's office	During and immediately after skill-learning session	Audiotaped role play with practitioner; rating forms; self ratings	Listening to tape; reviewing client's and practitioner's ratings
6. Practice in discussions with practitioner	Practitioner; two other practitioners	Practitioner's office	During and immediately after skill practice	Videotaped role play with practitioner; rating forms filled out by all practitioners; self ratings	Watching tape; reviewing client's and practitioner's rating forms
7. Practice in discussions in daily life	Significant others	Home and work	During interactions with significant others, week of 3/4–3/11	Rating forms filled out at end of day by client and significant others	Practitioner collecting rating forms and reviewing them with client at end of week

that Paul was unable to practice listening successfully to the other person's side in discussions in daily life. Thus, the practitioner knew that Paul needed a modification in order to help him learn this skill. The practitioner modified Paul's program using both approaches. In modification 1, the practitioner revised the listening practice step and redeveloped a program to meet this new subgoal. In modification 2, the practitioner added a new step to the original program in order to facilitate the practice of listening.

Practice Situations

Assume that in monitoring Mary's progress you have discovered that she is unable to complete a step in the program. Using a format similar to that depicted in Table 50, write two modified programs for Mary using the modification approach discussed earlier — that is, revising a step and adding steps.

SUPPORTING THE CLIENT'S UTILIZATION OF THE COMMUNITY RESOURCE: A SUMMARY

Goal: To ensure that the program to utilize the resource is implemented and that the community service coordination effort is successful

1. Develop time lines for action.
2. Develop reinforcers to ensure action.
3. Develop a monitoring plan.
4. If necessary, modify the program to improve its effectiveness.

Table 50. Program Modifications (Paul)

Steps in Disagreement Program

Modification 1:   Revising a step

New Subgoal: Practice listening to other's side in discussions in daily life (originally step 7*b*)

	Starting Date	Completion Date
Practice in discussions with strangers:		
a. Practice with the bus driver	3/9	3/9
b. Practice with clerk in grocery store	3/10	3/10
Practice in discussions with significant others:		
a. Practice with close friend	3/11	3/16
b. Practice with mother	3/13	3/16
c. Practice with coworker	3/15	3/16
Practice in discussions with others:		
a. Practice with others at home (family, friends, neighbors)	3/17	3/20
b. Practice with others at work (coworkers, supervisors, boss, customers)	3/20	3/23

Modification 2:   Adding steps

New Step: Practice listening to conversations on radio or TV

a. Develop a practice schedule	3/4	3/4
b. Practice paraphrasing brief comments (ten words or less)	3/9	3/11
c. Practice paraphrasing longer comments (over ten words)	3/11	3/13
d. Practice paraphrasing comments of two speakers	3/13	3/18
e. Practice paraphrasing each comment of one speaker for entire half-hour	3/18	3/19

107

SUPPORTING THE CLIENT'S UTILIZATION OF THE COMMUNITY RESOURCE: A SKILLED APPROACH

Joyce walked briskly into Richard's office, looked directly at him, and said, "Hello, Richard, how are you today?" Then, a bit sheepishly, she said, "How's that for being assertive?"

"Great," Richard laughed. He took pleasure in her confidence, yet he was aware how fragile it was. Joyce's life for the past years had been a pendulum of hospitalization, attempts at independent living, and re-hospitalization. She would attain a degree of stability that she couldn't sustain outside an institution. The basic but numerous tasks of every-day living at some point would overwhelm her.

In his years as a rehabilitation practitioner, Richard had come to see how community resources could be used to help clients develop the ability to live independently. More importantly, Richard had learned that his responsibility did not end or diminish once a referral was made.

Joyce and Richard had agreed that Joyce would initially remain in the hospital and attend the Berkshire House day program, where she would learn basic skills vital to independent living.

"I want you to describe our plan for the next few months, OK?" Richard said.

"OK — for the first month I'll attend the day program at Berkshire. I'll get there by bus. I'll work on housekeeping tasks, balancing a budget, using free time constructively. The next month I'll move into their residency program."

"And . . ."

"And, you and I will meet every Wednesday, and you'll contact the director of Berkshire House every Friday to discuss my progress."

"Right. Don't forget though, Joyce, this program can be modified. If you have any problems, if any difficulties arise, you can have additional time to learn a specific responsibility."

Before leaving, Joyce turned at the door. "I want to thank you. I think this time I can make it."

As she left, the door swinging behind her, Richard thought, "This time, with ongoing support, we'll stop that pendulum."

Chapter 5 EVALUATIONS AND APPLICATIONS OF COMMUNITY SERVICE COORDINATION

EVALUATING THE EFFECTIVENESS OF COMMUNITY SERVICE COORDINATION

The basic *outcome* measure for community service coordination is whether the client actually utilizes the resource and attains the desired referral goal. Attainment of the referral goal is, of course, highly individualistic and varies with the specific benefits the client is to derive from the resource being used. For example, a client working through an employment service might be expected to obtain a job, hold the job for a year, be satisfied with the job, and earn a certain amount of money. Through the use of a transitional facility, the client might be expected to make a satisfactory adjustment to an independent living situation.

Outcome measures thus focus on the ultimate benefits obtained by the clients through the use of community resources. To evaluate outcome, then, the practitioner will want to set operationalized referral goals and follow the client to assess the degree to which the goals have been achieved.

In addition to outcome measures, evaluation can focus on *process* measures. Process measures can essentially be defined as the interim behaviors or skills that facilitate the achievement of the desired outcome. With regard to community coordination skills, these process measures can focus on the practitioner or the client.

At the practitioner level, one area of process evaluation is the degree to which the practitioner can articulate the rationale for the selection of a particular resource. Community resources should not be selected without a well-defined rationale. In other words, the practitioner should be able to articulate: (1) one or more referral goals that are to be accomplished by the resource; (2) the alternative resources that were considered; (3) the client values used to evaluate the alternatives; (4) the relative importance of different client values (i.e., their weights); (5) the amount of each client value that was considered very favorable, favorable, and so on; (6) how well each alternative measured on each value; (7) how the alternatives should be ranked relative to the other resources in their ability to satisfy the client's values; and, if needed, (8) additional alternatives developed by modifying or generating new alternatives. In short, the evaluation focuses on whether the practitioner can present a comprehensive decision-making model based at least in part on the client's own preferences.

A second area of process evaluation at the practitioner level is the degree to which the practitioner can articulate a plan for utilization of the resource. In other words, the practitioner should be able to specify any of the following: (1) the agreement-negotiation steps needed to obtain the resource's commitment to helping the client; (2) operationalized client problems that might interfere with the successful use of the resource; (3) operationalized resource problems that could reduce the effectiveness of the resource's efforts with the client; (4) the current client and/or resource functioning in the problem area; (5) the desired level of functioning in the problem area (i.e., goal); (6) the steps necessary to reach the goal; (7) time lines for when the steps will be taken; (8) the differential reinforcements that will be used to facilitate the client and/or others taking the needed steps; (9) the monitoring steps that will be used to determine the progress of the implementation of the program; and (10) the ways in which the program can, if necessary, be modified. In summary, process measures at the practitioner level focus on the degree to which the practitioner makes a systematic decision concerning which resource to use and then develops a comprehensive plan to use the resource effectively.

These same process measures can be used at the client level. The determination as to what level of skill development would be appropriate can be based on the functioning of the client. High-functioning clients might be expected to be able to articulate the decision-making process and their part in the implementation plan. Low-functioning clients might be expected to articulate the referral goal, the next step to be taken, the time line for accomplishing the step, and what reinforcements (if any) will be forthcoming for completing or not completing the step.

Whether the process evaluation is for the practitioner or client, the approach can involve a straightforward questioning procedure. For example, the practitioner might be asked to show how she or he arrived at a decision to use a particular resource. Scoring would then be done by checking to see what decision-making components were present in the process. By the same token, a low-functioning client could be asked, "What are you trying to accomplish with the resource, and how will you do it?" Scoring would then be based on whether the client could articulate the goal to be accomplished at the resource, the next step to be taken, when the next step would be done, and what would be the consequences if the step was or was not completed.

Collection of data for process evaluation may follow either written or oral procedures. With practitioners and high-functioning clients, written evaluation is generally best, because the skills in coordinating community resources are too complex to be presented easily at a verbal level. Of course, one need not have a separate test for practitioners. Where community resources are used in the rehabilitation process, the practitioner's case records can simply be examined. With low-functioning clients, especially if reading and writing are a problem, an oral question-and-answer approach will be more effective.

It should be pointed out that, in addition to evaluating practitioner or client functioning at the end of the rehabilitation process, the same questions can be used to diagnose practitioner strengths and weaknesses in the area of community service coordinating skills *prior* to hiring the practitioner; likewise, similar questions can be used to diagnose client strengths and weaknesses in regard to using community resources *prior* to the commencement of the rehabilitation process.

With the practitioner, such a diagnosis will help the agency to know the level of functioning possessed by a particular candidate for a job. The diagnosis can be used to make determinations about hiring and about the specific areas where a new practitioner will need in-service training. With regard to clients, such a diagnosis will let the practitioner know about the client's strengths and weaknesses in making use of community resources. For example, the client who is clear on his or her goals and can articulate the steps for using a resource is a very different client from the one who has no idea about what she or he wants from community resources or the steps to be taken to utilize them. This pretreatment diagnosis, combined with a posttreatment evaluation, will provide a pre-post assessment of progress that can serve as a process evaluation measure for the practitioner.

To summarize, the effectiveness of community service coordination skills can be evaluated with both outcome and process measures. The process evaluation will identify the extent to which the skills involved in the effective coordination of community resources are being used. The outcome measures will identify the benefits that accrue to the client. In general, then, the process evaluation of community coordinating skills will focus on the practitioner, and the outcome evaluation will focus on the client.

APPLICATIONS OF COMMUNITY SERVICE COORDINATION SKILLS

The presentation of the skills in this book has followed ًstep-by-step developmental approach to community service coordination. That is, the major skills have been ordered so that they reflect a logical sequence in which a practitioner would take a client through all the phases of community service coordination, as illustrated in Table 1, Chapter 1. However, in addition to presenting a comprehensive model of community service coordination, this text has also attempted to teach a number of discrete skills that the practitioner can use as the need arises. These skills relate directly to the many different roles in which a practitioner must function: diagnostician, resource person, decision maker, coordinator, advocate, negotiator, program planner, support person, and monitor. The community service coordination specialist (e.g., case manager, coordinator, community support worker) functions at times in almost all these roles. The discrete skills presented in this text as part of the entire community support coordination model help facilitate the practitioner's ability to function in each of these roles, as the particular need arises.

Table 51 is a repetition of the presentation in Table 1 of the stages and skills of community service coordination. In addition, Table 51 shows how each of these skills relates to a role often required of the practitioner. Obviously, the skills do not fit discretely into these roles. The purpose of Table 51, however, is to show how mastery of the various skills of community service coordination helps to prepare the practitioner to function in a number of different roles.

As was mentioned in Chapter 1, not all of these various skills are used with every client. For example, in using the decision-making skills the practitioner can simply be guided by the principle that systematic decisions are necessary when (*a*) there is more than one community resource to consider; (*b*) there are several values or criteria to be considered; (*c*) no one alternative is clearly more favorable; and (*d*) the decision is important. In summary, the practitioner need use formal decision-making skills only where she or he feels it will functionally contribute to community coordination.

In summary, all the community service coordination skills presented in this text should be used only when and if they are needed to help improve the client's community functioning. The entire sequential model of community service coordination has been presented as a guide to facilitate the comprehensive learning of these skills. A highly skilled community service coordinator (e.g., case manager) will have most of these skills in his or her professional repertoire. In each unique client situation, the practitioner will draw on those skills most helpful to that particular client's community resource needs.

Table 51. The Stages, Skills, and Roles of Community Service Coordination

Stage I. Selecting the Appropriate Community Resource

Skill	Role
A. Identifying the client's community resource need	Diagnostician
B. Identifying available community resources	Resource person
C. Identifying viable resource alternatives	Diagnostician/resource person
D. Understanding the client's values and preferences	Diagnostician
E. Researching the potential resource alternatives	Resource person
F. Choosing the appropriate community resource	Decision maker

Stage II. Arranging to Utilize the Preferred Resource

Skill	Role
A. Preparing to make the resource aware of the client's need	Coordinator
B. Obtaining the agreement of the resource to provide service	Advocate
C. Finalizing the arrangements to utilize the resource	Negotiator
D. Developing a program to utilize the resource	Program planner

Stage III. Supporting the Client's Utilization of the Resource

Skill	Role
A. Developing time lines for action	Program planner
B. Developing reinforcers to ensure action	Program planner/support person
C. Monitoring performance	Monitor
D. Modifying the program to improve its effectiveness	Program planner

DATE DUE

DEC 1 '81 AB 16 '82			
MR 04 '85			
GAYLORD			PRINTED IN U.S.A